Applying Ancient Wisdom to Today's Food

Scientific evidence and Ancient wisdom

Dr. Deepa Bhargava

Cover designed by Kamlesh Bhargava

Dr. Deepa Bhargava

First Printing: February 2019

The information contained in this book is not meant to take the place of medical care under the direct supervision of a doctor. It is not intended to diagnose, treat, cure or prevent any disease. It is meant to supplement the advice of your personal physician, whom you should consult regarding individual medical conditions. Before making any changes in your health care, consult a suitably qualified doctor

About the Author

Dr. Deepa Bhargava MBBS, MS. is an Integrative Medicine specialist (Integrative medicine is an evolving form of health care where alternative therapies are integrated with conventional care) She based in Ontario Canada and is a member of the American Association of Integrative Medicine and the Canadian Integrative Medical Association.

For 35 years practiced as a senior ENT surgeon with a sub specialization in pediatric ENT, was also a senior teaching faculty member in a medical university tertiary care teaching hospital in Oman. She is passionate and has always believed in the philosophy of integrative medicine. For the past 34 years, has cared for thousands of patients by integrating surgery, medication, best of natural therapies, mind-body medicine, and Herbal medicine along with other natural solutions. She has been a lead researcher, and has published over 60 research papers, including several book chapters and books.

Some of her latest books are "Medicinal Herbs and Spices Scientific evidence and Ancient Wisdom", "Intermittent fasting with herbs and spices Current evidence and Ancient wisdom.

About the Book

The reason I have written this book is that I am convinced that today most of the chronic illness we are suffering from like Obesity, diabetes, heart conditions, Alzheimer's, Dementia, Arthritis, auto immune disorders are due to chronic inflammation at cellular level. Nutritional insights good as well as harmful have a huge role to play in reversing or managing these conditions. There is a need for everyone to understand how food can positively and negatively impact our health. For this we need to understand the science of Nutrition, science of the Microbiome and the effect it has on the genes and ultimately our health.

Today what we end up eating is influenced by many factors some being, personal preferences, social, political, economic, physical, metabolic factors and lastly the most important our dwindling cultural influences. Nutrition-related chronic disease conditions due to tissue inflammation, can be controlled to a large extent by the food choices we make. Its surprising to realize, today far more people are dying due to toxic lifestyle, which leads to Obesity Diabetes, Heart disease, Stroke, and many more chronic degenerative diseases as opposed to natural calamities, war or terrorist attacks combined.

What this generation has done to food since the Second World War is just appalling. Ancient time's culture and tradition taught people how to eat, preserve and sustain themselves, as we have progressed and advanced socially, economically we have also succumbed to many influences in the name of modernization. Culture, tradition and wisdom with food have slowly become very rare and forgotten to a larger extent, but the good news is slowly we are awakening to the ancient wisdom with today's food.

Finally we are seeing light at the end of the tunnel. While I was still writing this book, the new Canada Food guide published 22 Jan 2019 pleasantly surprised me. The food guide has incorporated all the current best scientific evidence, to make recommendations. It's very interesting to see they have recommended plant based eating, mindful eating, eating home cooked meals and preserving cultural food traditions. What is very impressive is they have kept the health of Canadians as a priority, ignoring the fact that the recommendations are bound to hurt the Food Industry.

This book is a step forward as it takes the reader to the scientific cutting edge of "personalized nutrition". Besides wisdom from latest cutting edge science this book is about personalized nutrition the future of personal health care, as the "one size fits all" approach is no longer effective. Its focus is on simplified practical action for strengthening the Microbiome along with the support of macro and micronutrients.

It is for those who want to educate and empower themselves with knowledge to improve self-care, prevent diseases, heal their bodies naturally, prevent or rid themselves of chronic diseases. For the modern fast paced life this book presents how you can develop a personalized   plan to incorporate this knowledge and wisdom in a simple easy to follow plan. You need not buy any expensive products most natural health products are available at your grocery store if not your kitchen!
For many it may be a missed opportunity as it's going to be years before this wisdom reaches the health providers and common man.

The first chapter reveals the truth of what you are really eating, it explores the latest scientific epigenetic and Neutrigenomic effects of today's food on health.

In the second chapter the reader learns about the basic building blocks of our food; the macronutrients that is about carbohydrate, protein and fat. The importance of micronutrients is discussed along with basics of the Vitamins, minerals and other micronutrients.

The third chapter reveals the current scientific communities focus of attention "the relationship of food with the Microbiome, Probiotic and Prebiotics". Science has identified that ones, microbiome may be a primary factor determining your health and longevity. Armed with this knowledge you can really make a difference to your health.

In chapter four the book reveals knowledge and secrets from *Ayurveda* 'The Ancient Wisdom of centuries. The combination of wisdom from latest scientific research and Ancient practices offers the reader an opportunity for personalized cellular and genetic healing possibly more than any expensive medication.

In chapter five and six we move from knowledge to action; the reader can develop an action plan for navigating the dilemmas of eating in the present food world of abundance. You can develop a personalized plan based on your specific health conditions to achieve optimal health.
Lastly in chapter seven the reader can enjoy Ancient Wisdom recipes for successes in your journey to good health.

CONTENTS

INTRODUCTION

Hope is nature's way of enabling us to survive
So that we can discover nature itself
Swami Dayanand Saraswati

What we end up eating is influenced by many factors some being, personal preferences, social, economic, physical, metabolic factors and lastly the most important our dwindling cultural influences. Today nutrition-related chronic disease conditions continue to be an issue. If not all, most chronic diseases are due to tissue inflammation, which can be controlled to a large extent by the food choices we make.

What this generation has done to food since the Second World War is just appalling. Since Ancient time's culture and tradition taught people how to eat, preserve and sustain them. As we have progressed and advanced socially, economically we have also succumbed to many influences in the name of modernization. Culture, tradition and wisdom with food have slowly become very rare and forgotten to a larger extent, but the good news is slowly we are awakening to the ancient wisdom with today's food.

Nutritional insights good as well as harmful have a huge role to play in reversing or managing chronic disease conditions. There is a need for everyone to understand how food can positively and negatively impact our health. For this we need to understand the science of Nutrition, science of the Microbiome and the effect it has on the genes and ultimately our health.

Most mainstream doctors have been trained to diagnose and treat disease symptoms; we have no doubt of the expertise of scientific mainstream medicine in diagnosing chronic problems and managing acute problems and disease. However when it comes to prevention, reversal of chronic disease conditions like Hypertension, Obesity, Diabetes, Coronary Heart disease, Allergies, Arthritis and most autoimmune conditions they are both deficient and incomplete. The main reason for this is a lack of understanding and accepting the power of nutrition. In my own experience after 32 years of practicing, researching and teaching medicine, I felt I knew nothing of healing, role of nutritional management, it is only after experiencing a great impact of this management, with transformation of my own health, my patient's health lead me to a sabbatical on epigenetic and Nutrigenomics' this book is a result of this research, education and experience.

This book explores this wisdom predominantly from Ayurveda, an ancient over 3000 years old system of Holistic natural healing that has its origins in the Vedic culture of India. This system was lost during foreign occupation, but is now enjoying resurgence globally the science of nutrition is very new in contrast to the wisdom of Ancient culture, however the prestige of science is much more than that of culture. This book covers wisdom from the latest scientific evidences in Nutrition, Nutrigenomic science, and relevant research on the Microbiome.

The initial chapters provide an overview of Today's food, its effect on your health and the science of nutrition, especially the micro biome. Subsequent chapters move from knowledge to action basically developing a personalized nutritional plan. Finally there is a section on some recipes for success

History of food, and Diets

Mankind has been struggling to make right food choices since time immemorial –A wrong food choice by Adam and Eve in 0BC –and here we all are!

Historically in Ancient times man ate whatever they could gather and hunt, most of the time this couldn't have been much and a lot of time and energy would have been spent on obtaining food and nourishing themselves. As we started to evolve the earliest agricultural revolution started so our food consisted of what we could grow, harvest store and consume; this mostly was grains, vegetables and fruit. We also started raising animals. It was not very easy to do all this a lot of crop was destroyed by pests, animals died of diseases and also in those times man succumbed to communicable diseases mostly infections. The food was pure, wholesome, and natural in this phase, however it was in small quantities so there was no need of any diets.

Then next phase in food history was of " the great agricultural revolution" pesticides were discovered to protect the food supply from pests, antibiotics were a blessing as they not only increased the life expectancy of man but also increased the life span of farm animals. Since we started to see abundance of food along with it came non-communicable diseases like Obesity, heart diseases, arthritis, and other inflammatory diseases.

The next phase in the history of food demonstrates the greed of mankind; the phase of the Genetically Modified Food and mass Animal farming, on one hand and on the other hand was the large food corporations marketing the processed food. The major supply of today's food no longer resembles what it originally was, most of today's processed food besides GMOs has additives like monosodium Glutamate to increase the foods palatability and crave ability. To increase the shelf life preservatives are added. Taste, cravability, longer shelf life, conveniences, commercial profit became a priority for the big food companies.

Along with all these convenience food, fast food, culture of dining out, luxury in the name of modernization came chronic diseases especially obesity, gradually more than 60% of population in developed world became obese. As a result many diets arrived; 1930 the ginger fruit diet, 1950 the cabbage soup diet, 1955 fast food diet, 1963 Weight watchers, 1985 Fit for life, 1988 Oparahs liquid diet, 1989 saw the height of the low fat diets, 1992 we saw the food pyramid, 1994 The Atkins diet, 1995 the Zone diet, 2000 the macrobiotic diet, 2003 the south beach diet, 2010 The Paleo diet, in 2015 we saw the High Fat diet and in 2017 the Ketogenic diet. However nothing seemed to work and non-communicable diseases continued to increase by leaps and bounds.

With dismay many of us are a witness to the fact that the food supply, nutrition advice, even medical advice to some extent is all channeled to grease the wheels of the Capitalists. The food lobby and pharma lobby became very powerful and influential. Dietary guidelines got influenced non-communicable diseases continued to increase at a faster rate.

Finally we are seeing light at the end of the tunnel. I was pleasantly surprised by the new Canada Food guide published 22 Jan 2019.While I was still writing this book had to delay the book publication to incorporate discussions on the guide. The food guide has incorporated all the current best scientific evidence, to make recommendations. What is very impressive is they have kept the health of Canadians as a priority, ignoring the fact that the recommendations are bound to hurt the Food Industry.

Summarizing the Canadian Food Guide January 22 2019

Guideline 1 recommends

Nutritious foods are the foundation of healthy eating; Vegetable, fruit, whole grain, protein food should be consumed regularly among the protein food; plant-based protein food should be the choice these protein food include legumes, nuts seeds, tofu, fortified soy beverage, fish, shell fish, eggs, poultry, lean red meat including wild meat, low-fat milk, low-fat yogurts, low-fat kefir and cheese lower in fat and sodium.

Foods that contain mostly unsaturated fat should replace foods that contain saturated fat.

Water should be the choice beverage.

Guideline 2

Processed or prepared food and beverages that contribute to excessive sodium, free sugars or saturated fats undermine healthy eating and should not be consumed regularly. People are encouraged to consume home cooked meals.

Guideline 3

Food skills are needed to navigate the complex food environment and support healthy eating.

Cooking and food preparation using nutritious food should be promoted as a practical way to support healthy eating.

Food labels should be promoted as a tool to help Canadians make informed choices.

The guideline also encourages developing healthy eating habits - healthy eating is more than the foods you eat it's also about where when why and how you eat. The guide advises on mindful eating; be mindful of your eating habits take time to eat notice when you are hungry and when you are full. More often plan what you eat involve others in planning and preparing meals enjoy your food culture. The guide also advises keeping food tradition alive as it can be part of healthy eating, it advises eating meals with others.

We whole-heartedly support the new Canadian food guide as the recommendations are Evidence Based, Unbiased, practical and a huge step in health management for the Canadian population.

Future of Food and Nutrition

Personalized Nutrition

The future is the era of personalized Nutrition. Research has shown every one processes macro and micronutrients differently. Often people are in situations that every food choice is a nightmare especially people with Insulin resistance. Can personal nutrition help people achieve their goals? The goals could be as simple as increased eating confidence in social and emotional situations, eating comfort, and weight loss. The goals could be as complex as wanting to reverse autoimmune disorders, heart disease or arthritis. We all would like to know what food is right for us, we all would like to know how to navigate ourselves through the thousands of food choices, identify an ideal meal. We all want the confidence that every food we eat is nutrient dense and is just right for us.

Nutrition is an important risk factor for metabolic disease especially for diabetics, and obese people that would mean more than half of world's population. The one-size fits all approach are bound to fail. Recent research has shown that the glycemic response of food is partly governed by the Microbiome this explains why the blood sugar response of different people to identical meal is so different. What this means is general diet advised to populations has a limited efficacy. The future lies in personalized Nutrition.

Personalized Testing

An era of Microbiome movement is around the corner. Microbiome testing and management is the future of nutritional science and medicine

Nutritional testing –measures body's actual level of vitamins, minerals and nutrients necessary for bodies proper functioning. Blood, urine, saliva, stool, hair nails are sent for analysis. Nutrigenomic testing of genes related to nutrient, metabolism, cardio metabolic health, weight management, food intolerances is rapidly developing and evolving.

There is a whole range of technology available at a steep cost for those who can afford. Those who can implement the recommendations in a disciplined manner are bound to benefit. However the technology is still evolving. Mainstream cannot adopt these as full scientific validation and approval is awaited.

Today's food tribes

Today the world has become divided in food tribes this is criticized by the establishment.

Actually deep down humans have a tendency to belong to tribes?

According to a 2014 fact report: 44% of adults admit food restrictions, food allergies, avoiding certain ingredients that dictate what they eat.

2015 NBJ special Diet Report mentions five dominant food tribes: gluten free, paleo, vegan, vegetarian, and raw vegan. This is probably not a bad thing as these individuals are possibly highly tuned to their bodies and have studied the effects of food on how they feel. In the future with personalized nutrition getting more popular these tribes will be accepted.

Why do we need Ancient wisdom?

Ancient wisdom has evolved over a period of thousands of years of observation. The basic Ayurvedic wisdom is based on practicing elimination and addition, on the philosophy of; "let your body do the talking". Based on this philosophy the practitioners, studied the detailed effects of various foods on subjective and objective health outcomes. Although it may seem inaccurate to many, the fact that it has survived through centuries cannot be ignored.

We all have heard a simple but powerful statement" we are what we eat". Another one is "Let food be thy medicine "as Hippocrates said. Ayurvedic wisdom is in harmony with these statements.

Scientific evidence is slowly and steadily validating these Ancient statements. We need to recognize the true power you have over your own health; your health is not like your age as your age continues in one direction only whereas your health is dynamic you can be young and in poor health and old and in good health.

What are your plans for the future? Do you wish to live a life disease free, never to be diagnosed with cancer, not to fall victim of diabesity, hypertension, heart disease and arthritis?

Applying the wisdom passed on from ages to your health can be one of the greatest gifts you can give to both yourself and your loved ones.

Let me warn you at times the information presented may not only be shocking but also depressing, however it will be worth it.

Would not go into statistics of the global pandemics of ill health facing us, but would like to stress how serious this situation is with today's food. Our hope is that by shining a light on the reality of this situation, you will be able to recognize our food supply and take steps to prevent further damage and take steps to reverse it before it is too late.

Today's food is nothing like what our ancestors ate the list is;

- Genetically modified pesticide laden fruit and vegetables
- Genetically modified grains wheat, soy, corn and rice
- Eggs from poultry raised in cages, fed GMO grains and raised on hormones and antibiotics
- To add insult to injury the Food processing industry has highly processed the food. Food is designed in laboratories with so many additives a long list some being Monosodium glutamate, preservatives, high fructose corn syrup and many more that we don't even recognize.

It is sad and depressing to see that our food is fighting a losing battle; against poor quality mineral and micronutrient depleted soil, GMOs, pesticides toxic farming practices, toxic food processing and marketing practices.

Can go into details of each of the above listed food items but then the focus of the book will be lost. Our focus is the basic knowledge to develop our own customized action plan so that our health and families benefit from applied knowledge of this Ancient wisdom and scientific evidence.

Food and culture

If we studying cultures for food wisdom we observe that many cultures have successfully learnt how to eat less by navigating the food jungle e.g. the Japanese. They have kind of mastered the art of eating ; their food is fresh, minimally processed, mostly plant based, in small quantities, they eat till 80 percent full, they need to be mindful while eating and it is a cultural tradition to drink tea eating is a very social and cultural event for the Japanese.

Similarly Middle Eastern cultures have a lot of wisdom too, the Mediterranean diet is one of the healthiest diet this fact has been validated by research too.

Similarly the Vedic culture has a lot of wisdom to offer this is mentioned in the chapter on Ayurveda.

Our health care needs a revolution

Due to Standard American Diet (SAD), most of us have got into the Sugar, Caffeine, Chemicals, Alcohol, and Nicotine, addiction and habit without being aware of it. Today far more people are dying due to toxic lifestyle, which leads to heart disease, diabetes, obesity, stroke, and many more degenerative diseases.

It's time to start tuning our lifestyles and learning what is best for us so that we can have better and optimum health leading to increased health span.

Are you are ready to transform your life? You are about to embark on a journey that will give you profound results possibly more than any expensive medication

As the Information age grows with leaps and bound there is bound to be allot of confusion, but we must not forget the Ancient wisdom about food.

With the increasing popularity of integrative medicine the concepts of personalized nutrition is rapidly gaining popularity and will be an integral part of healing in the future decades. As the information age continues to leap forward, it is bound to confuse and complicate the practice of medicine. Informed patients will be searching for therapeutic options, particularly for conditions where conventional approaches don't work. In countries where governments fund health care, patients will demand a broader spectrum of researched options to manage their care, including epigenetic intervention, neutrigenomic-based management, supplements, and herbal products. Already the science of lifestyle Genomics has been introduced and hopefully will gain popularity in future. Sadly however for many who are ignorant of this knowledge it will just be a missed opportunity!

There is, therefore, a critical need to reformat medical education to train providers in integrating alternative medicine. Hopefully in the future the complex mind, body, and spirit interplay would be better understood, so that these interventions are available to impact the healing of the body.

If you want to improve your self-care, prevent diseases, heal your body, rid yourself of diseases you should educate and empower yourself with latest knowledge. This will be your first step to healing nutritional management.

During the journey of writing this book I learnt a lot from my research on today's food and ancient wisdom. The solutions you'll find in this book are based on published clinical research, and Ancient wisdom derived from careful observation accumulated over almost a period of 10000 years. They are also based on my own journey of explorations dealing with my own health challenges and healings with my patients. I now eat a lot of local organic whole food plant based food, eat a variety of food including fermented food, supplement with minerals and vitamins. Have rediscovered the benefits of Ayurveda and vedic lifestyle; disciplined Vedic diet, Yoga- meditation, gratitude, sleep etc. Have thoroughly enjoyed the journey and transformation with my health. My sincere hope is that this book will provide you with solutions that will help you reclaim your energy, health and vitality, setting you on a disease-free path.

CHAPTER 1.
TODAY'S FOOD AND ITS IMPACT ON OUR HEALTH.

The way we live, along with our nutritional practices is probably the most powerful tool we have when it comes to protecting our health. We need to reexamine and consider how modern life and our everyday choices affect us.

If you think you already lead a healthy lifestyle and feel great, you'll be surprised how most of us have gotten used to being fatigued, bloated, and inflamed with food intolerances, allergies, gastrointestinal aliments like gassiness and many more illnesses. We live in a world where people are increasingly getting disconnected to their bodies

Historically our ancestors not only survived but also thrived by; eating simple food offered by mother nature this nourished them sustained them. They ate fresh unadulterated local fruit, vegetables, eggs, dairy, naturally processed oils. They maintained their health and were protected from many of today's chronic disease like Obesity, diabetes, heart disease and cancer to name a few. Unfortunately they did succumb to infections.

Then things started changing – more food was needed so farming began over the next 10,000 years farming evolved into a profitable business and industry. In the history of mankind the last 20 years will be remembered as a period where we have witnessed a detoriation of our food right from the seeds to our table. Today's food is very different from the food consumed by our ancestors. The present day food has very little in common with the food of our ancestors just 200 years ago.

Recognizing today's food

Today's food is nothing like what our ancestors ate the food is 80%Genetically Modified Organisms (GMO) the genetic modification of organisms is conducted in laboratories. Genes are artificially inserted from bacteria, viruses, insects, animals or even humans into the DNA of a food crops or animals in order to make them; increase yield, reduce maturation time, heartier to withstand weather changes and improve resistance to pests. As per current statistics 80% of packaged food in the United states contain GMO, 94% of soy, 90% canola, 88% corn,100% beets, 80% Hawaiian papaya, and 25 thousand acers of zucchini, peppers, tomatoes, squash are grown using GMO seeds, it is surprising that still 20% of our food doesn't contain GMOs.[1]

The list of GMOs is

- Genetically modified pesticide laden fruit and vegetables
- Genetically modified grains wheat, soy, corn and rice
- Genetically modified vegetable oils heated denatured and hydrogenated creating poisonous trans fats
- Eggs from poultry raised in cages, fed GMO grains and raised on hormones and antibiotics.
- Milk from genetically manipulated cows, raised on hormones, antibiotics GMO Grains. The milk itself is pasteurized with many additives.

- Meat laden with antibiotics, hormones from animals caged and raised on GMO grains
- Genetically modified Fish raised in tanks and fed GMO pellets.

A lot of processed food is created in the lab coming to think of it, it is not real food but a product which labeled as food e.g cheese slices, artificial meat and so many more.
It is sad and depressing to see that our food is fighting a losing battle; against poor quality mineral and micronutrient depleted soil, GMOs, pesticides toxic farming practices, toxic food processing and marketing practices

To add insult to injury the Food processing industry has highly processed the food. Food is designed in laboratories with so many additives a long list some being Monosodium glutamate, preservatives, high fructose corn syrup and many more that we don't even recognize.

We are increasingly disconnected from our food and bodies. We have outsourced cooking to the industry without even realizing it. We mostly eat at restaurants, fast food joints, take away and buy packaged food. Very few of us have the time, inclination to put in effort, or skills to put into home cooking. This is understandable, as the outsourced food tastes way so much better and is really enjoyable besides being so convenient.

Would not go into statistics of the global pandemics of ill health facing us, but would like to stress how serious this situation is with today's food. Our hope is that by shining a light on the reality of this situation, you will be able to recognize our food supply and its effects on your health, and take steps to prevent further damage and take steps to reverse it before it is too late.

A growing food movement is afoot, people are awakening to the fact that we need to recognize our food today the food is very opaque and it's also invisible to us. We hardly know where our food comes from, who grew it, how it was sent and how it was given to us, the industry prefers us to be in this state, and they don't want us to see how it's produced. You will be surprised that it is a criminal offence to photograph farms. This is probably because they don't want any one asking uncomfortable questions.

Today the food chain is very long globalized, economically driven one. We have lost control over it. The saddest example of this is in Europe a beef burger was discovered with many different kinds of meats one of them being horsemeat! Historically another example is mad cow disease as cows were being fed cows. Seriously this should have been a learning moment .The food industry just wants you to keep consuming food in a packages so that the wheels of capitalism keep getting greased. We like it too as it is cheap, convenient tastes excellent. Wonder how many of us realize have just been tricked. We really need to pay attention to where the food is coming from.

A positive fact however is an alternative food market the organic movement and the farmers markets are growing. It's nice that today there are some people who are ready and don't mind paying more for food which they know, how it is grown, and from where it is coming from. If we want to see any success in the food movement globally we need to get people off the processed food.

Poor quality topsoil produces food lacking in micronutrients

Another important fact is that the soil quality has detoriated and it's quite alarming that the food of today, fruits and vegetables lack minerals and vitamins. Farmers are being pushed, for economic reasons to grow crops faster, the focus is on breeding high yielding crops that can withstand natural adversities these genetically modified Organisms GMO varieties form the foundation of today's food.

What is very disturbing now is the quality of the earth's topsoil. Now it takes far more fertilizers to produce the same amount of food and the produce lacks in the micronutrient as has been abused for a long time and its quality has substantially deteriorated. The soil lacks in minerals, vitamins, valuable bacteria and other micronutrients due to over farming and neglect. One of the reasons for this is also mono farming as for economic, political and commercial reason all we like to grow is wheat, corn and soy. An ancient farming wisdom has been rotating crops as when we grow legumes it enriches the soil with nitrogen. Another ancient wisdom practice was animals grazed in the farm and manure was naturally produced this enriched the soil with microorganisms and nutrients, but now animals are confined to pens. To add insult to injury soil is laden with pesticide to get larger amount of food. Because of all the chemicals we are putting on the soil the bacterial life of the soil is threatened. The natural logic of biology and the logic of industry are in deep conflict. Unfortunately all this means our food is lacking in micronutrients and as the logic of industry wins biology loses we are facing an epidemic of non-communicable diseases like diabetes, obesity, and autoimmune disorders.

There is a serious need to reunite the animals with the farm currently the animals are sitting in the feedlots this practice has led to multiple problems sick animals' infertile soil and finally sick of human beings. There is a serious need to restructure the agriculture.

Pesticides and Herbicides in our food supply

Some GMO crops have been genetically engineered not to i.e. when sprayed with the Glyphosate herbicide (Round up). The way Glyphosate works on the weed is by latching onto, chelating the essential minerals they need to survive. Round up is the most used and abused weed killer it is destroying the soil, reaching the drinking water supply. Glyphosate is the world's bestselling herbicide used in 90 countries and on more than 150 crops. The crops have been engineered to withstand Glyphosate but the animals, fish and human's health suffers as it leads to micronutrient deficiency, ultimately effecting the epigenetics.

It's very disturbing to realize this chemical is hiding with the GMOs in every aisle of our grocery store. 2

Factory farming and our Global Food System

In 1945, 40% of all vegetables consumed in USA were grown in backyards[3]. In contrast today most of our food is produced in factory farms, often traveling a great distance before reaching our tables. The USDA estimates 39% fruit, 12% vegetables, 40% lamb and 78% fish and shellfish are imported each year from other countries. 4   Another statistics is; in the last 50 years world's population has doubled however the food shipped between countries has quadrupled. All this has affected the quality of food in terms of its micronutrient levels; as the vitamins suffer due to exposure to different temperature during transportation, also premature harvesting of fruits and vegetables prevents them from obtaining optimal micronutrient levels. How often have we bitten into a beautiful perfect fruit to be disappointed by its flat taste in terms of flavor, sweetness or tartness? This is often because of the above farming techniques so always try to eat local and seasonal.

Farmed Animals instead of Farm Animals

In the name of advancement and the fact we live in a capitalist society raising of farm animals has also changed. Did you know?

90% of salmon served in USA is factory farmed. [5] The fish are farmed in aqua farms, often sea lice is a problem due to overcrowding, Salmon are carnivores but these fish are fed food pellets packed with GMO corn and soy. The result is sick fish, micronutrient deficiency and low omega -3, [6].

Cows are supposed to eat grass but now cows are no longer roaming free they are caged together in pens and are fed on a diet of genetically modified corn and soy. Now also they are fed stale chocolate and candy. The beef from these cows is artificially high in fat, low in minerals vitamins and other micronutrients.

Chickens are worse off as they are caged and eggs produced are nutrient depleted[6]
The worse practice however is that the animals are given antibiotics to increase body weight and hormones to mature faster more on these in chapter on Microbiome.

Food processing

Identifying heavily processed food is easy it comes in a box, bag, or bottle. These foods have been engineered to be convenient, palatable, addicting, and poor in macronutrients, poor in micronutrients. They have a high crave ability index. too!!

Milk processing by pasteurization robs its micronutrients. Additives like carrageen are added all this kills the friendly bacteria.

I wonder if you know that the fruits and vegetables are irradiated to increase the shelf life. This is a harmful practice as it kills friendly microbes that are essential for our Microbiome. Irradiation destroys vitamins, minerals, and essential fatty acids. Since the shelf life is prolonged in the end all we get is empty calories.

During my research was surprised to learn that anything we do to our food depletes its micronutrients in some way. Even slicing, dicing, peeling, sautéing, cooking, baking, and microwaving exposes food to air, light or heat. All this depletes the micronutrients.

In Chapter 5 and 6 we will give you details of how to navigate the food industry for protecting your health.

Menacing Monosodium Glutamate (MSG)

MSG is really a menace it works in three ways; it intensifies the tastiness by dilating the taste buds, it makes you crave more of the treat as it causes insulin spike, leading to more hunger, it blocks Leptin which is the hormone that makes you feel full. So the food industry simply loves MSG as it can get population addicted, coming for more and their cash registers keep ringing by the sales.

MSG besides being an excitotoxin can cross the blood brain barrier; overexcite cells cause brain damage, worsen learning abilities, Alzheimer's disease, Parkinson's disease, Lou Gehrig's disease. MSG also places demands on our valuable micronutrients causing them to be depleted. So you can see it is one of the worst antinutrients of our food supply.

Personally I have been very interested in MSG as I am severely intolerant to it, even small amounts in my food lead to crippling Migraines. In my food intolerance journey have really researched MSG to my dismay have discovered MSG has many names the food manufactures have been out to fool us, many aliases of MSG exist; Glutamate, Glutamic acid, Magnesium glutamate, Mono ammonium glutamate, Monopotassium glutamate, Natural flavors, Sodium caseinate, Soy isolates, Soy sauce, Vegetable extract, Carrageen, Autolyzed yeast, Yeast extract, enzyme modified food and flavor enhancer are some aliases of MSG. It's lurking not only in processed food, fast food, and restaurant food and in most of the store bought seasonings too.

The Epigenetic effects of food on our Health

Genomics is the study of the genes as a dynamic system over time, determining how they interact and influence biological pathways, networks, and physiology, in a global sense.

There is an epigenetic basis for health and wellness. All your cells are genetically identical but structurally and functionally different due to the exposure of the genes and the interactions between the genes with our environment. Gene –environment interaction, especially the genes of the trillion microbes triggers almost all human diseases. Gene methylation and histone modification play an important role in the development of disease and in the aging process. So you can see how external environmental influences like diet, toxins, nutrients, and many more factors influence your Microbiome, epigenetic process and produce a state of disease.

Modern Science is now slowly discovering ways to   reverse the gene expression; the major way is paying attention to the Microbiome, paying attention to macronutrients, micronutrients and our food in general.

Nutrigenomics links to our food

The link between food and health is well documented, but people still are continuing to search for the right balance between energy intake and energy expenditure in order to prevent disease and promote a healthier lifestyle that meets cultural and genetic needs.

Nutritional genomics, or nutrigenomics, is the study of how foods affect our genes and how individual genetic differences can affect the way we respond to nutrients (and other naturally occurring compounds) in the foods we eat.

Currently, nutrigenomics is receiving research attention because of its potential for preventing and treating chronic disease and certain cancers through small but highly effective dietary changes.

The basic principle:

The degree to which your diet influences the balance between health and disease may depend on your genetic makeup.

Under certain circumstances, your diet can be a serious risk factor for the occurrence of a number of diseases. e.g excessive sugar and carbohydrate leading to diabetes.

Some diet-regulated genes are likely to play a role in the onset, progression, and severity of chronic diseases like obesity, diabetes, heart disease, and arthritis

Some dietary chemicals can act on the human genome, either directly or indirectly, to alter gene expression or structure. Currently there are hundreds of artificial chemicals from pesticides to preservatives in processed food, which we are ingesting, and these are interacting with our gene expression. In fact blood from the umbilical cord of unborn babies has shown these toxic chemicals.

How food can affect us negatively

The leaky gut

Your digestive tract is a hollow cylinder from the mouth to anus. In a healthy gut the food ingested is digested, macro and micronutrients are absorbed and the bodies nutritional needs are met and one remains healthy. In many of us the inner lining is damaged due to; disturbed Microbiome, overgrowth of yeast like Candida, parasites, harmful bacteria, toxic diet rich in sugar, refined carbohydrates, chemicals, gluten, alcohol, medication and many more substances.

In this situation the guts lining is no longer a barrier to these toxins, which freely enter the blood stream and this leads to body inflammation the cause of most chronic diseases. It leads to food allergies, autoimmune disorders and many other diseases.

Food intolerances

So now it's no secret that in the present modern day we all live in a toxic environment. We can acquire toxins from our environment, by breathing them, ingesting them or being in physical contact with them e.g. Most drugs, pesticides in food, chemicals for processing and preserving food, fertilizers remnants in food products, food additives, Monosodium Glutamate, GMO food, artificial sweeteners all can create toxic elements from reactions and by products in the body, these unstable molecules are also called free radicals. When these biochemical toxins are not counteracted or eliminated they inflame the cellular tissues this leads to cellular death, tissue degeneration presenting as chronic disease like Hypertension, Obesity, and Diabetes, Arthritis etc.

With time the bodies' detoxification mechanism gets affected

Detoxification is an integral cellular mechanism that is ongoing at microcellular level the toxins in the body are eliminated to the tissues, via the blood stream to the liver where the toxins are eliminated in the bile to the intestines, the skin, kidneys and the colon also are important organs which help in eliminating the toxins.

To some extent the normal young healthy body is able to rid these substances from the cells with the help of antioxidants, robust excretory system of the liver, intestines and kidneys. The liver plays an important detoxification role, however as we age these natural mechanisms get fatigued, clogged and inefficient. As a result of this, these toxins start getting accumulated. Most dangerous impurities and chemicals are stored in our visceral / abdominal fat, slowly this fat gets pro-inflammatory and starts wreaking havoc; affecting the basic hormones and messing up your body's metabolism. The first thing to be effected is the ability of the body to process sugars, this leads to impaired metabolism of heart, and pancreas. Visceral fat is a key factor; it releases an abundance of free fatty acids and increases the hormone Cortisol. The fat goes to all organs, causing inflammation. The abdominal fat cells are not just passive fat cells; they secrete many harmful hormones (adipokines), which worsen Insulin Resistance.

Insulin resistance and its effects

Insulin resistance (IR) is one of the most pressing problems in the developed world today.

IR is the cause of metabolic syndromes which have the following characteristics: abdominal obesity, hypertension, elevated lipid levels, especially triglycerides, low-density lipoproteins (LDL, the bad guys), and reduced high-density lipoproteins (HDL, the good guys). People suffering from insulin resistance are at risk of developing platelet dysfunction, heart attack, stroke, cardiomyopathy, sleep apnea, polycystic ovarian syndrome, Non Alcoholic Fatty Liver Disease, liver inflammation, or cirrhosis.

For an insulin sensitive person, insulin works efficiently to manage the glucose from our food so that the pancreas secretes the proper amount of insulin to clear glucose from the blood stream. However, in a person with IR, insulin is rendered ineffective and it cannot enter the cells. As a result, the pancreas produces more insulin to push the insulin into the cells for energy expenditure. Insulin stimulates the conversion of glucose to fat. So the root of most chronic illnesses today is insulin resistance. The cause of insulin resistance is both genetic and lifestyle related.

Lifestyle factors are the major factors:

The Standard American Diet (SAD) a high carbohydrate, toxic, and inflammatory diet, is the major cause of IR. Lack of exercise is the second contributing factor. Stress and emotional distress also are known to complement IR. All these lead to a vicious cycle of sugar cravings and emotional eating.

The key is maintaining metabolic balance by maximizing nutrition and minimizing the impact of toxins.

How food can affect our health positively

For food to have a positive impact on our health we need focus on personalized nutrition (more on this in chapter 5 and 6), eating according to our nutrigenomic profile, and paying attention to our Microbiome . Dietary interventions based on knowledge of nutritional requirements, nutritional status, and genotype (i.e., personalized nutrition) can be used to prevent, mitigate, or even cure chronic disease.

Currently tests are available to test analyze and recommend the suitable eating pattern the science is still evolving and has not yet been approved by FDA so your mainstream doctor will not recommend it if you request testing. However some of the positive effects of the right type of food on your health are mentioned. By applying the Ancient wisdom coupled with personalized nutrition you can achieve optimal health.

Taking care of leaky gut

For this you need to have a clever gut diet as Hippocrates said" All diseases begin in the gut" Taking care of your Microbiome is the key to taking care of the leaky gut more in next chapter on this. Thanks to today's food most of us need supplementation by probiotics, prebiotics or symbiotics.

Eating the right type of food can slow and reverse our aging

Science is beginning to show that the main causes leading to shortening of the telomeres besides aging are lack of nutrients in food, stress, toxins, and lack of exercise. All this at cellular level leads to degeneration and aging of the cells. This is also responsible for most diseases. Most of the present day chronic diseases result from clogged tissues, suffocated cells causing loss of vital energy. So if you would like to get younger or improve your health span you can choose to detoxify, pay attention to diet and supplement diet.

Curb unhealthy cravings and storage of abdominal fat.

Most of the chemical toxins are fat-soluble and are stored in abdominal fat. Since these chemicals are fat-soluble our bodies gets the message to consume more fat to dilute these chemicals and get rid of them. Most of the fat is metabolized by the liver, which is mostly not functioning well in overweight people so the fat ends up getting stored in abdomen. Abdominal fat is a factory for harmful hormones, which greatly harm most of our body organs including heart and brain.

Aim for Sustained Weight Loss

Eating the right type of food coupled with Cleansing supports the bodies' ability to loose pro inflammatory "stubborn fat" can lead to weight loss. The fasting regimes often lead to autolysis (breaking down fat stores of the body for energy). The herbal supplements prevent formation of free radicals, neutralize existing free radicals and finally reduce oxidative stress all this leads to healing process at cellular level. Finally this leads to sustained and maintained weight loss.

Improve Digestion

By incorporating high fiber intake you can improve digestion; Excessive mucus, bile and waste from the digestive tract are expelled with the fiber; fiber helps bowel movements improve with a relief from excess bloating and gas. The consequent healing of the gut leads to many health benefits and healing at many organ and cellular level.

Improve Liver functions

The liver suffers the most from poor quality food exposure and excessive alcohol. The liver is responsible for detoxifying the body internally. The liver is where dangerous toxins are metabolized so when healing of liver functions happens due to detoxification many health benefits are experienced.

Boost Metabolism: With improved nutrition body will be able to digest foods at a more efficient rate with improved metabolic functions. Benefits of boosted metabolism are

- Boosted vitality and energy levels are the rewards of improved metabolic functions by consuming the right kind of food.

- Increases Mental Clarity: By improving nutrition many people feel as if "a fog has lifted." Not only do they get more energy but they also think faster, clearer and keep their focus for longer.
- Improved Sleep: Improved digestion and the right type of food can lead to a better night's rest and sleep.
- Improved Skin Health: Many people have food intolerance once identified and eliminated can lead to beautiful, blemish free radiant skin. This is the first sign of removed toxins.
- Emotions: Positive healing effect on the emotions. Many people notice that detoxifying heals emotional issues.

Future of Nutrition and Medicine 2050 And Beyond

- The prediction is food will be a huge political and social agenda. Trade agreements may get abandoned.
- Global population and global trade will continue to grow.
- Climate changes, along with increased pressure on natural resources will be a worldwide issue
- Higher food prices with increased household expenditure predicted.
- Quality fresh foods will be available to those who can afford them.
- Clean Plant based Food will be valued and animal protein will be reduced considerably

References

1. Nongmoproject.org/learn more/what is gmo.
2. Nongmoreport.com/articles/consequences of widespread Glyphosate use.
3. Yesmagazine.org/issues/can animals save us/ Joel Salatin –how to eat meat and respect it too.
4. Ers.usda.gov/media/157859/faul125 pdf.

5. FDA.govt/Advisory Committees/Committees Meeting Materials.
6. Farmed Salmon and human health. Pure Salmon Campaign; pursalmon.org/human health.
7. Food irradiation and human health.

CHAPTER 2.
FOOD MACRO-NUTRIENTS AND MICRO-NUTRIENTS

"When it comes to obtaining the micronutrients your body needs, your best possible source is food, especially fruits and vegetables. But circumstances may prevent you from eating optimally every day. The main reason I take nutritional supplements is for insurance against gaps in my diet. I take supplements faithfully and encourage my patients to do so as well."

Andrew Weil, M.D.

You are what you eat, and every day science is proving the validity of this powerful statement.

Everyone knows about calories, Food macronutrients- Carbohydrates, Protein and Fats. Generally everyone is familiar with micronutrients too – Vitamins, Minerals, and many more health enhancing micronutrients present in supplements. These are not the focus of the book, the focus is today's food and how to navigate to obtain optimal health. However we discuss these powerful building blocks of our bodies.

Macronutrients

The three macronutrients or macro for short are carbohydrates proteins and fats they are the three suppliers of energy in our diet and support most of our bodies' vital functions.

Carbohydrates

They are the main composition of food and provide energy in terms of mental and physical activity they are simple carbohydrates and complex carbohydrates.

Simple carbohydrates are

- Monosaccharide's which the main components are, these are found in glucose fructose and galactose. Glucose is the regular sugar, fructose is fruit sugar and galactose is the milk sugar.

- Disaccharides are sucrose and lactose
  Simple sugars come in the form of products containing refined carbs like bleached flour, sugar sweets or candy sweet, soft drinks and fruit juices containing high fructose corn syrup these should be avoided at all costs.

Complex carbohydrate

Fiber and starch are complex carbohydrates.

- Polysaccharides are the complex carbohydrates: Amylopectin that is plant starch and Inulin these are very important these days for an healthy Microbiome.

- The sources of complex carbohydrate include vegetables, fruits, legumes, cereals and grains, sweet potato, whole grains, brown rice and many of the ancient grains: Buckwheat, Sorghum, Amaranth, Millets, Finger millet, Fox tail Millet are some ancient grains, they are very precious and most beneficial form of grains that you could use.

- The Glycogen is carbohydrate that is stored in the body it is mostly stored in skeletal muscle that is 2/3 of the carbohydrate, 1/3 is in the liver your glycogen stores provides you with energy during physical activity and every time the stores are replenished when you eat a meal which is rich in carbohydrates.

- The ancient wisdom has always been to favor the complex carbohydrate whenever possible. Now modern science is discovering the health benefits of the complex carbohydrate.

1. Complex carbohydrates do not lead to sugar spikes which simple carbs can lead to.
2. Additionally complex carbs keep you fuller for a longer time as they have a strong dose of fiber.
3. They are rich in minerals and have a positive effect on your intestinal Health on your microbiome.
4. Complex carbohydrates have been shown to help lower the cholesterol levels.
5. Currently a lot of attention is being focused on prebiotic. Actually the benefits of prebiotic food was known to the ancient people it is basically the food which contains fiber the indigestible carbohydrate this acts as a source of nourishment for the microorganisms that live in the colon of the body the common sources of prebiotic are: legumes, artichoke, rolled oats and different fibers we talked about the probiotics we have covered in length in the next chapter.

Proteins

The next group of macronutrients is the proteins; proteins are made up of link chains of amino acids.   The human body contains 20 different amino acids basically the amino acids are divided into three categories the essential amino acids the semi essential amino acids and the non-essential amino acids.

We are incapable of producing sufficient essential amino acids before we have to be sure that we are getting this from our diet some of the essential amino acids are valine, leucine, isoleucine, histidine, lysine, methionine, and tryptophan.

- Some semi essential amino acids are; glutamine proline tyrosine glycine and taurine.
- The non-essential amino acids are alanine, aspartic acid, glutamic acid.
- The protein component of macronutrients does a variety of jobs in the human body; it helps make the hormones, enzymes and antibody in the human immune system.
- Proteins also are a part of certain body's structures like connective tissue the muscle fiber skin hair is all made out of proteins, 60% of the body's protein is stored in the muscles your protein source do not serve as a direct source of energy but work like building blocks for other structures of the body.
- The recommended dose for protein in the diet is one gram of protein per kilogram of your body weight on a daily basis if you are looking to build muscle mass you can increase your intake and take the 1.2 to 1.22 grams per kilogram body weight. Professional athletes and those who are doing intense exercise can aim at a post workout meal in the ratio of 1 is to 3 carbohydrates. This protein ratio helps with muscle growth and leads to anabolic effects of this hormone
- The high protein foods that you could have are eggs, meat, fish, seafood, milk and other dairy products. The vegan sources of protein are nuts, seeds, legumes, grains and some vegetables. Studying ancient cultures and their traditional food revealed a lot of wisdom its amazing how they combined grains, legumes and vegetables to achieve benefit of all the amino acids.

Fat

Fat the flavor carrier is an important macronutrient in the diet it has been demonized in the past but is now slowly gaining more popularity as new evidence appears about its benefits.

- Every cell has fat, it is needed to regulate the metabolism and also maintain the elasticity of the cell membrane.

- Unsaturated fats also improve the blood flow and are very important for cell growth and regeneration.
- The fats just don't provide the body with valuable fatty acid they also deliver the fat soluble vitamins like vitamin A, D, E and K.
- Fats provide the human body with cholesterol, which is synthesized through the exposure of sunlight to form vitamin D in the skin.
- Fat is also important for hormonal production.

Fat comes in different forms:

1. Saturated fats: Saturated fats comes in solid form like butter, coconut fat, fat that is present in meat, meat products, and dairy products.
2. The monounsaturated fat these are in olive oil, flaxseed oil, avocado oil, and nut oils. These fats have a lot of health benefit can help with weight loss, reduce risk of heart disease and decrease body inflammation.
3. Trans fats - trans fats are those fats which have been heated once, following this they're made solid by a process and these are present in the baked goods, fried food and some type of margarine that should be avoided at all costs because they're very damaging to the body. They cause inflammation at cellular level causing genetic degeneration.
4. Polyunsaturated fats -Essential fatty acids – are fatty acids that are essential for metabolic processes of the body and cannot be manufactured by the body. Omega-3 and omega-6 fatty acids are essential for the body good sources are cold water fish like mackerel, Herring, salmon and sardines are the richest form of these fatty acids. Flaxseed, hemp seed, olive oil, chia seeds, walnuts are other sources. Omega 6 is believed to be pro inflammatory, while omega 3 is anti-inflammatory. The ratio which they recommend to use is omega-3 and omega-6 ratio of 3: 1 currently people are consuming the ratio is 16: 1.

The basic message is all three macronutrients are crucial to your health and perform important functions in the body a balanced diet with the appropriate ratio of macronutrients is vital for staying healthy.

Micro nutrients

Micronutrients are a major group of nutrients which are essential for the body they include the vitamins, minerals and the other miscellaneous micronutrients that are being discovered every day.

Vitamins are necessary for energy production immune function blood clotting and many other body functions. Meanwhile Minerals play an important role for growth of bone, fluid balance and many more other processes of the body. Micronutrients have an immediate impact on our health to maintain your brain, muscle, bone health, nerve Health, skin, blood circulation and immune system our body requires a steady supply of vitamins and minerals. You only need a small amount of micronutrients failing to get a small quantity of this can lead to guaranteed disease.

The essential micronutrients are the 30 vitamins and minerals that your body cannot manufacture in sufficient amount on its own.

These include **vitamins, minerals** that you have heard about all your life and other less familiar substances — such as **herbals products, botanicals, hormones, amino acids, probiotics** and **enzymes**.

These micronutrients harness the inherent healing power of the body. A Variety of foods are important for a healthy diet, however supplements may assure that one gets an adequate dietary intake of essential nutrients.

Micronutrients have a significant role in preventing diseases, managing, healing chronic disease, and improving health and wellness.

Why have micronutrients not received their deserved popularity?

Modern mainstream medicine and its education have never truly appreciated the role of nutrition enough. Even though in the 19 th century major breakthrough dramatic cure discoveries of vitamin deficiency disease e.g Vitamin A curing night blindness, Vitamin D curing rickets, still role of micronutrients has been a forgotten science for researchers and doctors. Moreover till today it is unrecognized that a low dose deficiency state is very prevalent in society and this not only prevents optimal health but also is responsible for many chronic disease occurrences.

Historically there is convincing evidence that getting people to accept new medical ideas is very difficult. A classic e.g is when a British naval surgeon James Linde showed lime juice could cure scurvy it took 60 years for the medical community to accept vitamin C!

The medical establishment always insists on evidence based on double blind studies. Now which company will spend thousands of dollars on research on micronutrients that are natural occurring and which they cannot patent to reap a handsome financial profit.

Forgotten research: There are a whole bunch of studies that show the benefits of supplements, but there is no one to promote this evidence and bring it to the knowledge of practicing physicians, as a result if one were to ask his physician about vitamins the response one is most likely to get is "I'm not sure if it will help your condition, if you stick to a balanced diet you will get enough micronutrients"

In reality in 2014 there are 3 published studies that have shown: Adequate Vitamin D levels lower HbA1c in type 2 diabetes, low

Vitamin D status may be a risk factor for developing Alzheimer's and dementia and correcting low Vitamin D improves the severity of fatigue symptoms. .[1, 2, 3]

However your physician most likely is unaware of this new evidence, and probably will never know as no pharmaceutical representative is going to inform him about this as sales of Vitamin D does not get in much revenue.

Another factor is that most of the prominent Journals do not publish research on vitamins and supplements. So this research evidence has got forgotten to the advantage of the health care industry.

Today mainstream nutritional advice is dominated by the food industry, and pharmaceutical industry. This unfortunately means the information and advice is biased and can lead to a missed opportunity to optimal health for many of us.

What research says?

The research evidence on use of supplements is very flawed; firstly supplement sales don't generate a lot of revenue as compared to pharmaceuticals, so it is not in the interest of the health care industry to vigorously research them, secondly there is contradictory, biased evidence. All this has led to confusion within the health care community.

Most integrative practitioners with their years of experience support use of supplements.

Researchers have asked the question; does taking a daily multivitamin/mineral supplement really improve health? Unquestionably it does.[4]

Another study in 2003 looked at whether people who took a daily multivitamin/mineral had fewer infections than people who didn't. Researcher divided 130 adults into two groups one group took a daily supplement for a year and the other took a placebo. Nobody knew who got the real pill and who got the dummy. The study results showed only 43 % of those who had the supplement had infections like colds and flu whereas 73% of the placebo group got sick. Among the diabetic group 93% of placebo group got sick as compared to 17% of the supplement users. [5]

Still there is a paucity of research with reference to supplements. Hopefully this will change in future

The science of future

Nutrition, nutritional supplements will be a large part of medicine's future, supplement prescriptions already have become specialized, customized and individualized. Medicine is bound to get individualized already Genomic Lifestyle is being studied in detail and soon based on one's genomic legacy patient will receive Lifestyle and supplement recommendations. The next step to individualized medicine is Lifestyle genomics. It provides a framework to deal with one's genomic legacy for contributing to health and wellness.

Even today the Natural health product industry is a $40,000,000,000 industry with over 100,000+ available natural products in North America. However it is not well a regulated and monitored industry. At one end of the spectrum are mainstream practitioners who mostly are unaware of the mounting research on benefits of nutritional supplements and at the other end are the general population who are using supplements without knowledge of suitability, optimum dose and possible side effects. We recommend that you use supplements, after consulting with a knowledgeable healthcare provider first.

The list of supplements varies according to underlying conditions e.g there are different supplements for body builders who want to develop muscle mass, the list for you if you want to lose weight is different, similarly if one has   metabolic problems like high cholesterol, diabetes, heart conditions need a different set, people with immunological problems, arthritis have another specialized list. In this book we present a bird's eye view on basic supplements. Hopefully in future we plan to publish separate books for individual conditions.

With this newfound knowledge power, comes a community responsibility of sharing this with family and friends.

Aging and Telomeres what latest science says?

Telomeres are caps at the end of chromosomes it is a relatively new, important, and dynamic, Nobel Prize winning areas of aging science and medicine.

Length of telomeres is an indicator of biological aging. Telomere length at the ends is lost with each cell division. Dysfunction of telomeres is associated with aging and the development of many age-related diseases.

With aging after a certain number of cell divisions, telomeres in a given cell get critically short. Older people generally have shorter telomeres. Diseases, stress and a number of other conditions can also cause telomeres to shorten. Cells with too-short telomeres can die.

Science has revealed Telomere length is influenced by lifestyle including nutrition, oxidative stress, inflammation and activity of telomerase enzyme. Inflammatory processes that lead to repeat and increasing cell divisions lead to subsequent damage of telemetric DNA. In addition oxidative stress, reduced availability of nucleotide precursors, results in shorter telomeres.

Recent research has revealed; Anti-inflammatory and antioxidant nutrients can reduce erosion of telomeres. Nutrients also have the potential to influence regulation of telomere length, e.g., folate helps via its role in epigenetic status of DNA and histones, and nicotinamide helps through its role as a substrate for posttranslational modification of telomere associated proteins. Germ cells and stem cells express relatively high levels of the enzyme telomerase. Many normal body cells express little or no telomerase. Scientist have identified supplements that improve telomerase activity, a large privileged population is already happily consuming these supplements and experiencing health benefits.

Why do we need supplements?

- There are epigenetic factors, which alter the bodies' cellular metabolism; many of the supplements are needed at cellular level for optimal body functioning.
- Other toxins in the environment are pollution, pesticides, petrochemicals, electronic emanations – all increase our requirement of antioxidants to detoxify our system of this chemical burden, which damages our genes causing chronic diseases.
- As we age the cellular metabolic functioning gets sluggish due to supplement deficiencies.
- Though food may have been once sufficient, but today it is no longer so. The reason being the soil is depleted of nutrients.
- Several essential minerals have been depleted from the soil due to over farming e.g. Iodine depleted soil can be blamed for goiter and zinc depleted soil for premature aging heart disease and cancer.
- The food we consume has been processes, frozen, and overcooked. It has been estimated 80-90% of micronutrients of food is lost before we finally consume it. Even light steaming destroys nutrients.
- Refining of food is at the moment all-time high, this process turns the food into antinutrients. E.g. polishing of rice lead to beri beri. Refining depletes minerals like selenium, chromium, magnesium, zinc, manganese and copper.

- Sugar is an antinutrient however when consumed it needs to be metabolized and its negative effects on the body need to be counteracted to some extent.
- The mineral chromium is severely depleted and deficient this affects the sugar metabolism. I wonder if this is the cause of the global epidemic of obesity, and Diabetes.
- Lastly and most important most people today follow some kind of diet; calorie restricted, carbohydrate restricted or a fat restricted diet, this has a potential for developing micronutrient deficiencies.
- Virtually every study comparing supplement takers with a matched group shows that the group taking supplements is healthier.
- Research on Cancer patients has revealed that supplements used along with chemotherapy and surgery have reduced side effects, faster recovery, and improved survival

VITAMINS

Vitamin A

The skin protector and infection fighter. It was the initial infection fighter but now vitamin C has replaced it as the lead infection fighter. Vitamin A reinforces the immune systems resistance to infectious diseases, improves skin health, healing skin lesions and wounds, it has shown to improve pulmonary disease by improving the epithelium of the respiratory tract and prevents cancer. A recent study has shown that vitamin A helps stabilizing blood sugar in people with abnormal blood sugar. Children are particularly deficient in Vitamin A any child with recurrent childhood infections can benefit from vitamin A supplementation.

The adult dose recommended is 5,000 IU however for retinol deficiency states up to 100,000 IU per day may be needed.

Natural sources include: Cod liver oil, and liver are the best sources followed by butter, egg yolk, cream and whole milk.

Carotenoids, Beta – Carotene, Lutein and Lycopene

Are precursors of vitamin A however they have their own healing powers as powerful antioxidants. Research has shown that they have an important role in preventing and treating Cancers, heart disease and immune disorders. The natural source is colored vegetables and fruits like leafy dark greens, yellow, orange vegetables and fruit like beets, carrots, tomatoes watermelon and grapefruit. Strawberries though red don't contain it. It is important to remember if these sources are had, as a part of fat free diet the absorption is not satisfactory.

Vitamin B Complex

The energy givers. There are eight B vitamins
The B complexes are the nutritional key to vital body functions. The family includes B1, B2, B3, B6, folic acid, B12, Pantothenic acid and biotin.

<u>Vitamin B1</u> (*brain energizer*) the people who require B1 supplementation include older individuals, pregnant and lactating mothers, people with alcohol related cardio-myopathy, hypertensive's on diuretics, people with learning difficulties, emotional disturbances, Alzheimer's disease, neural disorders and pain.
Recommended dose is 50-100 mg. We need to remember although present naturally the vitamin is lost during cooking.

<u>Vitamin B2</u> (*antioxidant, energizer and team player*) Riboflavin has a role as a team player for many metabolic pathways e.g. its deficiency can weaken the thyroid gland. Critical illnesses elevate the need of B2

e.g. stroke, heart attacks, severe respiratory illnesses, also research has linked it to depression and other health problems. Dose recommended is 25-50 mg/day.

<u>Vitamin B3 Niacin and Niacinamide</u>   This is considered a "drug" and needs a doctor's prescription. Niacin helps reducing cholesterol and triglycerides, while niacinamide helps osteoarthritis and may prevent diabetes.
Dose: Niacin 100 mg to 1000mgms, Niacinamide 100mg- 300 mg. There are side effects so need to be used under medical supervision.
Natural sources include poultry, dairy products, seafood, nuts and seeds.

<u>Vitamin B6 pyridoxine</u> *the most essential B vitamin.* It is recommended for diabetes, heart disease, hormonal disturbances, immune weakness, Candidiasis, kidney stones, brain and nerve impairment, joint and hip pain and skin disorders.
Dose recommended is 25-100mgm daily

<u>Vitamin B9 Folic acid</u> (*the most vital vitamin*) prevents birth defects in pregnant women 4 mgs of folic acid daily can prevent 75 percent of birth defects. Useful for heart disease as it can correct high **homocysteine** levels a great risk for heart attack, stroke, Alzheimer's disease, multiple sclerosis, carotid artery stenosis, vein clotting e.g. retinal blood vessel leading to vision loss, menopause and peripheral vascular disease. The other recommendations are intestinal disorders, brain disorders like epilepsy, depression, cancer, skin problems it also has anti-inflammatory properties.
The chief dietary sources are liver, kidney, broccoli, beef, and dark green leafy vegetable like kale.
Dose recommended: 20 -60 mg per day.

<u>Vitamin B 12 Cyanocobalamin (*Vitality booster*)</u> Vegetarians, elderly, smokers, and people with chronic conditions are prone to B12 deficiencies. Helps improve mental function including a broad range of emotional and cognitive abilities, heart disease, multiple sclerosis, sleep disorders like insomnia, asthma and allergy, nerve pain, low blood pressure, viral infections, tinnitus, hearing loss, infertility and cancer.

Dose: 100 mcg every day. Higher dose recommended in disease states.

<u>Pantothenic acid:</u> Useful for balancing the lipid levels, soothing inflamed tissues in autoimmune disorders, cardiovascular disease, colitis, Chrons disease, yeast infections, gout, and obesity.

Dose 100-200 mgm daily higher doses recommended for disease conditions.

<u>Biotin:</u> Helps ensure skin and hair remain healthy, useful for managing Type 1 or type 2 Diabetes.

Dose: 5-15 mg with meals.

Vitamin C

It is a nutrient that is fundamental for each and everyone's health as it does it all.

Vitamin C is necessary for the body to form blood vessels, cartilage, and muscle and bone collagen.

It is particularly useful for colds, viral infections, all infections, cancer, high blood pressure, heart conditions, asthma, allergies, age related macular degeneration, atherosclerosis, stress, obesity, gout, gall stones, vision disorders, and drug addiction.

Dietary sources include citrus fruits, berries, tomatoes, broccoli and spinach. Don't forget Vitamin C is lost during cooking.

Dosage: For general health, at least 500 mg to one gm daily the natural sources are more potent than synthetic versions, divided doses are more effective. Also mixing with some minerals like magnesium and iron is useful.

Vitamin D

Your body manufactures vitamin D when direct sunlight converts a chemical in the skin to vitamin D. It is essential for building bones as the body can only absorb calcium when vitamin D is present.

The production of Vitamin D is dependent on: your skin color, where you live, lifestyle time of day, season (in winter in North America it is probably completely absent!)

Recent research has suggested that it helps prevent cancer of; colon, prostrate, and breast cancer. Older adults can reduce their falls by vitamin D supplementation. Vitamin D supplements prevent bone loss, osteomalacia, treats rickets. A topical preparation helps psoriasis. Also it is useful for improving sugar imbalance in diabetes, bowel aliments, multiple sclerosis, and arthritis.

Natural sources include milk and milk products, fatty fish and eggs.

Dosage: latest recommendation has increased to 1000 IU daily. Most people with chronic conditions may need a higher dose.

Vitamin E

Vitamin E exists in eight different forms. Its main function is protecting the body from free radical damage due to its antioxidant properties. It is useful for age related macular degeneration, Alzheimer's disease, cancer prevention and treatment, cardiovascular disease, neural impairment, immune weakness, blood disorders, menopausal symptoms, lung disease, immune weakness and arthritis. Natural source is vegetable oils and fats.

Dose: 400-1200 IU per day.

MINERALS

Potassium

Potassium is essential to managing blood pressure and is the most valuable electrolyte. Sodium raises your blood pressure. Potassium lowers it, may improve problems with kidney stones, and bone loss.

Dose: For most adults, the recommended daily amount is 4,700 milligrams (mg). Dietary sources are recommended. FDA has prohibited over the counter supply of potassium.

The best food sources of potassium are: Parsley, sunflower seeds, nuts, Avocados, Prune, and Tomato. You can also get potassium in chicken some fish, such as Halibut Tuna and Cod.

Bananas, Potatoes, Carrot, Orange and dairy products such as milk and yogurt also contain potassium.

Calcium

Your body needs calcium to help muscles contract and expand, blood vessels to stay healthy, to secrete hormones and enzymes and to send messages through the nervous system. It also helps in clotting blood; sending and receiving nerve signals, your body needs calcium to keep your bones dense and strong. Low bone density can cause your bones to become brittle and fragile. These weak bones can break easily, even without an obvious injury.

You have more calcium in your body than any other mineral. The body stores more than 99 percent of its calcium in the bones and teeth to help make and keep them strong.

Foods rich in calcium include: Dairy products such as milk, cheese, and yogurt, Leafy, green vegetables, Fish with soft bones, such as canned sardines and salmon, and tofu.

Dosage varies in different age groups: 800 mg to 1500 mg per day are recommended.

Magnesium

Magnesium is used in many biochemical reactions, like maintaining heart normal rhythm, immune system, and muscle function. Dietary sources include legumes, whole grains, nuts, and dark green leafy vegetables.

Research has shown low magnesium levels are associated with high blood pressure, diabetes, heart disease and osteoporosis. It also helps in reducing: attacks of migraine, mood swings in premenstrual syndrome, insomnia, and muscle cramps

Dose; 400-1000 mg

Zinc

It is a mineral found in every cell, and is essential for normal growth of cells.

Zinc is the immune booster and wound healer of the body, regulates appetite, stress levels.

Preliminary research has shown its benefits in sickle cell anemia, attention deficit/hyperactive disorder, neurological illnesses, diabetes, sexual health, and eating disorders.

Since the body is unable to produce zinc it can be obtained from diet: meat, fish, poultry, liver, milk, and wheat.

Daily dose: 15-25 mg. daily.

Copper

Both shortage and surplus of copper are harmful. It helps in heart function, controls cholesterol, sugar and uric acid. It also is needed to manufacture collagen in bone, is anti-inflammatory to bones so is useful for treating Rheumatoid arthritis. It is also immuno-modulatory. Dose- 2-3 gms only if indicated

Chromium

It is a trace element needed in small amounts needed for cellular functions. Research has shown that it interacts with insulin, so it probably helps in insulin resistance and appetite suppression.

Natural sources include seafood, green beans, peanuts and broccoli.

HORMONES AND OTHER COMPOUNDS

There is a very long list of compounds in this category but the scientific evidence of benefit is either not there or is conflicting, so only few are included.

Coenzyme Q10

Used to produce energy for the cell and has antioxidant properties. It is used to treat cardiovascular disease, congestive heart failure, statin induced myopathy, prevent aging and memory loss, to increase exercise performance, certain cancers. Also used in managing Parkinsonism, migraine, asthma, and high blood pressure. 150 -300 mgs.

Glucosamine and Chondroitin

Glucosamine and chondroitin are natural compounds present in cartilage. They are used to treat osteoarthritis. Glucosamine supplements are made from skeleton of shellfish. Choindroitin is made from shark and cow cartilage.

Omega 3 Fatty acid

Omega 3 fatty acids are essential for good health; they are derived from food and cannot be manufactured in the body.

Research has shown that it helps lower the risk of depression, improve brain health, improve cognition, improve cardiovascular risks like stroke, and improve symptoms of rheumatoid arthritis and osteoarthritis.

Side effects include increased risk of bleeding and depressed immune response.

S–adenosylmethionine (SAMe)

SAMe is a compound naturally occurring in the body. Its function includes production, regulation of hormones and maintenance of cellular membrane.

SAMe doesn't occur in food but a synthetic version is available. Recent research has shown it to be useful for managing depression, fibromyalgia, liver disease and osteoarthritis.

Drawbacks are its high price and has interactions with some drugs

PROBIOTICS AND PREBIOTICS

Technically, probiotics are not Miconutrients but are supplements. Prebiotics (oatmeal, flaxseed, onions, garlic, leeks, asparagus, and chicory roots) are herbal plant-based products. Both will be discussed below as currently are one of the most important supplement.

Probiotics

The World Health Organization defines probiotics as "live organisms, which, like bacteria and yeasts, when ingested in adequate amounts, exert health benefits in the host via the intestinal flora."

Probiotics are "friendly bacteria" that are similar to organisms that occur naturally in the digestive tract. Certain strains or types of probiotics have been linked to all sorts of health benefits, from helping with irritable bowel syndrome and traveler's diarrhea to boosting the immune system.

Normally, intestinal flora has more than 400 species of bacteria. It is recommended that for optimal health a ratio of 80:20, friendly bacteria to other bacteria, are needed.

This topic is discussed in detail in the following chapter.

HERBAL SUPPLEMENTS

This is a very wide topic with very exciting recent research findings pleases refer to the book "Medicinal Herbs and Spices Scientific Evidence and Ancient wisdom" http://www.amazon.ca/Herbs-Spices-Scientific-Evidence-Ancient-ebook/dp/B00J3CLPAU

References

1. Green RT, GambhirKK, et all. Maintenance of long-term adequate levels of Vitamin D Lowers Hb1Ac in African American patients with type 2 Diabetes. Ethn Dis. 2014; 24(3):335-41.
2. Thomas J. Littlejohns, William E. Henley, Iain A. Lang, Cedric Annweiler, Olivier Beauchet, Paulo H.m. Chaves, Linda Fried, Bryan R. Kestenbaum, Lewis H. Kuller, Kenneth M. Langa, Oscar L. Lopez, Katarina Kos, Maya Soni, and David J. Llewellyn. Vitamin D and the risk of dementia and Alzheimer disease. Neurology, August 2014
3. Ray S, Shuna A et all Correction of low Vitamin D improves Fatigue: Effects of correction of low Vitamin D in Fatigue study(EViDiF study) N AmJ Med Sic 6(8): 2014
4. Fletcher,R.H., Fairfield,K.M., Vitamins for chronic Disease Prevention in adults: Clinical Applications. Journal of the American Medical Association 287(23). 2002, 3127-3129.
5. Barringer, T.A.,Kirk, J.K., Santaniello, Ac ., et all Effects of a multivitamin and mineral Supplement on infection and quality of life. A Randomized, Double-Blind, Placebo- Controlled Trial. Annals of internal medicine. 138(5) 2003 365-371.

CHAPTER 3. UNDERSTANDING RELATIONSHIP OF FOOD, MICROBIOME, PROBIOTICS AND PREBI OTICS

All disease begin in the gut
Hippocrates
We all have an ecosystem of microbes that affect our overall health. Science has clearly shown how Microbiome, genome and nutrition are all interrelated they all need to be in absolute harmony with each other to keep us healthy. Any disruption in our microbiome, epigenetic and neutrogenetic environment can lead to health disruption and vice versa.

The Microbiome Kingdom

Think of the Microbiome as a complex rainforest. It throbs with life with millions and trillions co-existing organisms – bacteria, fungi, viruses and some protozoa. Together they form a wonderfully complicated eco system. There are more genes in our Microbiome then our human genes to simply put it we are more microbe than human.

Previously it was thought they have very basic functions: protect the gut from invaders, synthesize vitamins like vitamin K. Modern science has shown the amazing effects they have, some are;

Gene Modulation

We have only twenty three thousand human genes but have eight million microbial ones. The microbial genes signal the body genes to function well the essential functions like carbohydrate metabolism, detoxification, surprisingly our genome doesn't have this ability. This explains why inherited disease don't afflict a family members, the ones with a healthy microbiome are spared

Immune regulation

Our microbiome regulates our entire immune system. Exposure to a diversity of microbes is essential for a healthy immune system. Ultimately they govern the number of attacks of cough and cold that we suffer from, the range of allergic and autoimmune diseases we develop in our lifetime. A lack of good microbes can lead to an overactive immune system ultimately leading to auto immune diseases like: asthma, eczema, thyroiditis, diabetes, arthritis and most diseases due to inflammation.

Our microbes decide how much we weigh as they can decide how much energy our body can extract from the food we eat. They also control hunger signals, they control our cravings, and they decide the degree of blood sugar spike after a meal. Modern science is revealing weight loss is just not as simple as eating less and exercising more.

They not only protect our gut from invaders but also nourish it. The microbes don't have arms or legs but are excellent chemists. They take bits of food from the body to produce hormones and different chemicals. They convert sugars to short chain fatty acids, metabolize drugs, modulate genes, Neutralize cancer –causing compounds, synthesize B complex vitamins, synthesize fat –soluble vitamins like vitamin K and synthesize hormones.

They have a huge impact on our brains a very exciting area of biome research is the gut brain "psychobiotics" .The gut microbes can communicate directly with our brains via vagus nerve. They also produce neuro transmitters and hormones, which influence our behavior and cravings.

Messing up the Microbiome

Microbial disrupters are all around us – in the food we eat, the water we drink, cosmetics we use. A damaged microbiome along with genetic and environmental factors can create havoc with our health.

How the current modern life style has affected health.

Dysbiosis

Dysbiosis is a term that describes imbalances of good bacteria to bad bacteria. Currently almost every week there is new research findings blaming most medical conditions on dysbiosis. Dysbiosis is the root cause of common medical conditions like leaky gut, irritable bowel syndrome, autoimmune disorders, vaginal yeast infection and resistance to weight loss.

Recent research has also shown dysbiosis as a cause of many poorly understood symptoms; Food cravings, weight gain, bloating, gassiness, foul flatulence, rashes, food intolerances, fatigue, brain fog, feeling off, frequent infections and so many more.

There are many causes of dysbiosis, some major ones being a steady diet of junk food since child hood (details in next paragraph), taking antibiotics especially long courses like for acne, acid suppressant, steroids, anti-inflammatory drugs, birth control pills, alcohol, and stress.

The modern disrupters in today's food.

In the chapter 1 we have mentioned how our food supply has been messed up; GMOs, Factory farming, farmed animals, food supply channels, irradiation of food all are to blame as they rob us of the microbes.

The current life style has a detrimental effect on the human micro biome; there are a number of factors involved.

Use of **oral antibiotics** for infections: antibiotics have been very useful for treating bacterial infections and have been a boon to mankind they deserve credit for saving many lives. However over prescription and self-overuse is a known problem the antibiotics kill not only the harmful bacteria but also the health promoting friendly ones. [1]

The bigger problem with **antibiotics is use by the animal farming industry:** low dose antibiotics are routinely given to all farm animals to prevent infections as the poor living conditions of livestock make them prone to infections. [2]The magnitude of the problem can be estimated by the fact that 80 % of the manufactured antibiotics are consumed by the farming industry. Most people are unaware that a good portion of the antibiotics we consume is hidden in the meat produce that we regularly consume and this depletes our friendly bacteria in our gut.

Use of microwaves:

Microwaves are believed to sterilize the food bacteria bad as well as good. [3] In Ancient times there was **no refrigeration** nor microwaves so food cooked was kept out and this led to increase in probiotic content of cooked food by inevitable fermentation.

Processed food has a lot of additives and preservatives consumption of processed food can really disrupt our microbiomes. To improve shelf life of food stuffs like salad dressing, frozen foods, baked goods additive like polysorbate 80, lecithin, carrageenan, polyglycerols, and xanthan and other 'gums are added. Science has shown that chemicals in processed food can disturb the normal intestinal flora. In a study on mice these food additives were found to cause mild intestinal inflammation in a group of mice with normal immune function, subsequently in this group of mice this led to metabolic dysfunction leading to insulin resistance, hyperglycemia and obesity. In a group of mice with preexisting weak immune system these food additives led to chronic colitis with worse consequences.[4]

Artificial sweeteners have been blamed for damaging the microbiome by destroying and depleting the numbers of friendly bacteria.

Food additives such as these are all approved by the Food and Drug Administration (FDA), again highlighting the severe limitation of our current regulatory system. A study found that nearly 80 percent of the food additives approved by the FDA lack testing information that would help the agency estimate the amount people can safely consume before suffering health consequences.[5]

Other modern life practices like detergents, antiseptic use cleaning agents in the environment also has depleted the friendly bacteria along with the harmful ones there is need to discriminate and prevent overuse of these agents.

Fluorination and chlorination of the water is another issue. Basically anything, which kills the harmful bacteria, is sure to damage the friendly ones too.

Ancient wisdom: Historically How probiotics have helped health and wellness through the centuries?

Historically, fermented food has been a staple of people originating from all ancient civilizations. Even today in these societies traditionally they consume these probiotic rich foods daily. Let's look and study the microbiome enrichment practices of these ancient civilizations to extract the wisdom of centuries. Although this wisdom is not based on scientific research but has been based on years and years of experiences of generations the very fact that these practices have survived to the present day makes them invaluable.

The Belgians, noted for their longevity, consume a large amount of fermented milk called kefir. In fact Elie Metchnikoff who discovered this fact and described the benefits of *Lactobacillus delbrueckii Sub sp bulgarius* on the immune system and associated longevity he received Nobel prize for his work . In recent years, scientific studies have proven that kefir may help longevity and over all improved health. New research has shown heart disease, obesity, diabetes has its origins in inflammation. Probiotics like kefir help by stimulating the immune system.

The Koreans have a favorite, Kimchi that is made of cabbage, garlic, and a lot of cayenne pepper. Even after migrating to Western countries, most Koreans maintain the tradition of consuming kimchi for health and wellness.

Italians consume sauerkraut for health (currently this is getting popular with athletes and body builders).

In India, before a meal traditional people even today consume a glass of yogurt drink called Lassi (with live cultures), and a small serving of yoghurt after the meal. They also consume pickled and fermented vegetables with every meal. Indian cuisine has a big range of fermented food like Dhokla, Idlis, Dosas etc.

The Japanese have their own super food, Natto, Miso made with soya beans.

Most Asian and Mediterranean cultures consume pickled cabbage, eggplant, turnips, carrots, onions, cucumbers, peppers, besides Greek yoghurt and Lebeneh with each meal.

However as these societies are progressing and prospering financially, the spread of the so-called modern living is rapidly affecting their microbiome.

Probiotics are believed to be the future of medicine. The scientific community in general accepts that the gut microbiota composition and function can be regulated via probiotics

What is a Probiotic?

The World Health Organization defines probiotics as "live organisms, like bacteria and yeasts, when ingested in adequate amounts, exert health benefits in the host via the intestinal flora." [5]

The concept of probiotic was introduced by Nobel Laureate Elie Metchnikoff also known as the "father of Probiotics" In his publication the prolongation of life he mentioned significant health benefits could be achieved by ingesting these microorganisms. This led to the term "Probiotics"- meaning "for life"

There is a common misconception that all bacteria are harm full "germs". Probiotics are "friendly bacteria" that are similar to organisms that occur naturally in the digestive tract. Certain strains or types of probiotics have been linked to all sorts of health benefits, from helping with irritable bowel syndrome and traveler's diarrhea to boosting the immune system.

How do probiotics work and how do they benefit Human Health?

Both published research and clinical observations have contributed to health -promoting actions of probiotics: Probiotics maintain a balance between harmful and friendly bacteria, decrease intestinal inflammation by improving gut permeability they can lessen antigenic and allergic sensitization this can prevent auto immune disease. Probiotics also enhance local and systemic immune function. Cancer – chemo preventive effects of probiotics is being discovered too.

The World Health Organization has gone so far as to recommend the use of probiotic therapy (also called microbial interference treatment [MIT] as an alternative whenever possible[5]

Theories on the mechanism by which probiotics exert health benefits include:

- Stimulation of host immune response.
- Reducing the harmful bacteria in the gut, producing antimicrobial compounds that destroy or suppress the growth of harmful microorganisms.
- Competing with pathogens for the limited number of receptor sites and nutrients.
- Increasing mucin this blocks the adhesion of pathogens.
- Interference with bacterial toxins.
- Neutralization of dietary carcinogens.
- Modulation of cytokines and mediators
- Creation of a physiologically challenging environment for harmful bacteria e.g. low pH and producing toxic byproducts
- Prevent disease e.g. Faecalibacterium prausnitzii appear to play an important anti-inflammatory role in the human microbiota.

Normally, intestinal flora has more than 400 species of bacteria. It is recommended that for optimal health a ratio of 80:20, friendly bacteria to other bacteria, are needed.

Lactobacillus acidophilus is the most commonly probiotic bacteria. Lactobacillus, as the name suggests, has the ability to ferment milk sugar, lactose, into sour byproducts; these include lactic acid and hydrogen peroxide, which make the intestines and stomach an undesirable environment for disease-causing bacteria, like H. pylori, the bacteria that causes gastric ulcers. It is used to manage problems, including traveler's diarrhea and imbalances of healthy bacteria in the colon following antibiotic therapy.

L.bulgaricus is a lactobacillus species that ferments milk into yogurt, since it's not a normal inhabitant of the colon, its benefits disappear quickly when a person stops eating yogurt.

L. plantarum ferments cabbage to give sauerkraut its sour taste. It is normally a beneficial inhabitant of a healthy colon, so its benefits can persist for a long time after you eat sauerkraut. Lactobacillus supplementation decreases the incidence of colon cancer, infectious diarrhea, and food allergies. It also lowers cholesterol levels, and activates the immune system to ward off infections.

Bifidobacteria is the most common beneficial bacteria in the large bowel. Eating vegetable fiber, especially from asparagus, garlic, onion, and artichokes, favors the growth of bifidobacteria.

Saccharomyces boulardii is related to baker's yeast and is used to treat acute diarrhea caused by antibiotic use. Rarely, patients with mold allergy may react to it.

What Are Prebiotics, Metabiotics and Symbiotic?

These are also known as "probiotic enhancers" or colon food.

Prebiotics

Are precursors of probiotics, dietary fiber are the best source (oatmeal, flaxseed, onions, garlic, leeks, asparagus, and chicory roots) are herbal plant-based products`. Other sources of prebiotics are fruit, vegetables, wholegrain, certain fats, herbs, spices, red wine and dark chocolate.

Metabiotics

Scientists have discovered that even after killing the probiotic bacteria they continue to have health benefits as the bacteria's metabolic byproducts remain and serve as prebiotics some e.g short chain fatty acids like vinegar, butyric acid and propionic acid. All these are in fermented food like sourdough bread, Japanese Miso, Cheese, Indian idlis and dosas.

Symbiotic

Is both a probiotic and a prebiotic in a single product. Theoretically this combination should improve; microbial survival during transit through the upper digestive tract. Symbiotic stimulate metabolism and growth of friendly microbes within itself. It appears to be a interesting package deal unfortunately very little scientific data is available on Symbiotics, however many of the functional food ancient recipes described in the later sections are symbiotics.

How Safe Are Probiotics?

Probiotics by supplement or by functional food appear to be extremely safe[.3-5.].Caution is advised in following conditions: Immunocompromised patients, premature infants, Patients with central venous access and caution while using untested probiotic strains.[6]

Specific Medical conditions that have improved with probiotics

Antibiotic Induced Diarrhea:

Many meta-analyses have proven the benefits of probiotics. We now have scientific evidence of the benefits of probiotics, especially for antibiotic induced diarrhea [7]

Immune Function:

There's also evidence that probiotics help maintain a strong immune system. In societies with very good hygiene, we've seen a sharp increase in autoimmune and allergic diseases. That may be because pathogenic organisms aren't properly challenging the immune system. Introducing friendly bacteria in the form of probiotics is believed to challenge the immune system in healthy ways.[8]

Allergies:

Research also suggests consuming probiotics regularly may prevent allergies and eczema, and may also improve symptoms of lactulose intolerance.

Bowel Disease:

Probiotics can alleviate bloating and constipation, and generally treat inflammatory bowel disease.

Infections:

As probiotics boost the immune system, this can also reduce the frequency of infections and lessen cold symptoms. [9]

Heart Disease:

Probiotics may be helpful in lowering cholesterol and blood pressure.

Obesity:

Researchers are finding bacterial clues too, indicating these bacteria might be regulating how we harvest energy from our food. Two strains of bacteria have been found: *Bacteroiddetes* and *Firmicutes*. Lean people have more *Firmicutes* and fewer *Bacteroidetes*. Interestingly, it has been observed that as obese people lose weight, the ratio of friendly and not friendly bacteria also changes.10

Depression:

Deficiency of serotonin, an active neurotransmitter, has been closely linked to depression. Despite being called a neurotransmitter, 95% of serotonin is produced in the gut, with only 5% produced by the brain. The scientists refer to the gut as the "second brain." So by improving the gut function, deficiency of serotonin may be addressed.

Anxiety:

In patients with chronic fatigue syndrome, *lactobacillus casie* was found to significantly reduce anxiety symptoms. Probiotics can inhibit inflammatory molecules called cytokines, decrease oxidative stress, and balance the overgrowth of unwanted bacteria so that the intestines facilitate optimal nutrient absorption.

Recurrent urinary Tract Infections:

Probiotics have been shown to prevent recurrent UTI in women. Most of these women suffer from Vaginal Candida a fungal infection that makes the susceptible to the infections.

Other Benefits:

Though the research findings are preliminary, introducing prebiotics and probiotics together can have beneficial effects on aging, calcium absorption, even AIDS and type 2 diabetes. 11

Probiotics are generally regarded as safe and well tolerated. Some probiotics may be contraindicated in patients who are immunocompromised or have severe underlying illness, as they have been reported to cause fungaemia and bacteraemia.11

Fecal transplantation. FMT

While I believe fecal transplantation can be lifesaving in many circumstances like *Clostridium difficile*, Chrons disease, irritable bowel syndrome, ulcerative colitis and severe antibiotic- associated diarrhea. Currently more scientific support is awaited for use of FMT in Autism, Autoimmune disorders, Obesity Diabetes, Metabolic syndrome and Leaky gut.

If you address your gut health on a daily basis—by avoiding factors that kill off your beneficial gut bacteria, and continuously "reseeding" your gut through a healthy plant based diet and regular use of fermented vegetables, prebiotics, symbiotics and metabiotics you may never need one. Also, any time you take an antibiotic, it is important to take probiotics and/or fermented vegetables to repopulate the beneficial bacteria in your gut that the antibiotic kills.

References

1. Pharm M, Daniel A, Day AS. Probiotics Sorting the Evidence from the Myth MJA 2008;188:304-308

2. Huang JS, Bousvaros A, Lee JW, et al. Efficacy of probiotic use in acute diarrhea in children: a meta-analysis. *Dig Dis Sci* 2002; 47: 2625-2634.

3. Allen SJ, Okoko B, Martinez E, et al. Probiotics for treating infectious diarrhea. *Cochrane Database Syst Rev* 2004; (2): CD003048.

4. Jang C, Hui S, LuW, Cowan AJ et all Cell Metabolism Feb 2018 27,2:351-361.

5. Food and Agriculture Organization of the United Nations, and World Health Organization. Report of a Joint FAO/WHO Expert Consultation on evaluation of health and nutritional properties of probiotics in food including powder milk with live lactic acid bacteria. Cordoba, Argentina: FAO/WHO, 2001

6. Hempel S, Newberry S, Ruelaz A, et al. Safety of Probiotics to Reduce Risk and Prevent or Treat Disease. Evidence Report/Technology Assessment no. 200. Agency for Healthcare Research and Quality Web site. Accessed at http://www.ahrq.gov/clinic/tp/probiotictp.htm on May 10, 2011Prescribing Probiotics. Greenfield RH. In Integrative Medicine Rakel D 1094

7. Goldin BR, Gorbach SL. Clinical indications for probiotics: an overview. Clinical Infectious Diseases. 2008;46(suppl 2):S96- S100

8. Davidson GP, butler rn : Probiotics in pediatric gastrointestinal disorders Current Opin Pediatr 12: 477, 2000

9. McDade-Ngutter C, Versalovic J, Alexander W, et al. National Institutes of Health Gastrointestinal Microbiota and Advances in Prebiotic and Probiotic Research conference summary. Gastroenterology. 2009;136(5):1473-1475.

10. DiBaise, J.K.; Zhang, H.; Crowell, M.D.; Krajmalnik-Brown, R.; Decker, G.A.; Rittmann, B.E. Gut microbiota and its possible relationship with obesity. Mayo Clin. Proc. 2008, 83, 460–469. [

11. Food and Agriculture Organization (FAO) of the United Nations and World Health Organization (WHO). Guidelines for the Evaluation of Probiotics in Food. Report of a Joint FAO/WHO Working Group on Drafting Guidelines for the Evaluation of Probiotics in Food, London, Ontario, Canada, April 30-May 1, 2002. Accessed at ftp://ftp.fao.org/es/esn/food/wgreport2.pdf on November 4, 2011.

CHAPTER 4.
ANCIENT AYURVEDIC WISDOM

May the universe never abuse food.
Breath is food
The body eats food
The body rests on breadth
Breadth rests on the body
Food is resting on food.
The one who knows this
Becomes rich in food and great in fame.
Tattiriya Upanishad 11.7

Ayurveda medicine is one of the world's oldest holistic healing systems it was developed more than 3,000 years ago in India. Ayurveda is widely practiced in India today most of the Indians combine Western stream medicine with Ayurveda which is a legacy handed over from our ancestors.

The main principles of ayurveda are; the basis of everything is health and wellness, which depends on the delicate balance between the mind body and spirit.

When we go through classical Ayurvedic literature like *Charak Samhita, Susuruta Samhita, Bhavaprakasha, Charakadatta,* we will notice that ancient practices were much more advanced than we credit them for as they had a lot of food wisdom.

While writing this chapter have used the Sanskrit Ayurvedic terms, as a literal English translation cannot do justice to the essence of the terms. More over the relevance of the terms for readers from the Indian subcontinent will remain intact.

Ayurveda: A life Of Balance

Ayurveda is rooted in India's most cherished scriptures known as the Vedas, dates to about B.C 1500 – It's an ancient system of Holistic natural healing that has its origins in the Vedic culture of India. 1 Tibetan medicine and Traditional Chinese Medicine both have their roots in Ayurveda. Even early Greek medicine also embraced many concepts originally described in the classical ancient ayurvedic medical texts.

Although suppressed for centuries during years of foreign occupation, Ayurveda today has been enjoying a major resurgence in both India and globally. Currently Ayurvedic education has been formalized as a health care system in India. [2] Ayurveda is a science of life (*Ayur* = life,*Veda* = science or knowledge). It offers a body of wisdom designed to help people stay vital while realizing their full heath potential. A more precise translation of Ayurveda would be "the knowledge of the lifespan." [3]

Ayurveda offers practical tools, insights, and information for living in balance and health, without interference from illness. It reminds us that health is the balanced and dynamic integration between our environment, body, mind, and spirit. It is a healing system that treats the whole person – the integration of body, mind, and spirit – rather than simply treating individual symptoms. For example, we know that ongoing stress damages our immune system, and when the immune system is weakened, we are more vulnerable to disease and illness. Similarly we also know that when our mind experiences pleasure and happiness, our brain releases happy chemicals to our entire body, creating feelings of happiness and well-being this leads to healing at a physical level.

Ayurveda takes holistic medicine a step further, treating people not as isolated individuals but as an inextricable part of the environment and whole universe.

In India's ancient Vedic tradition, there is an underlying intelligence that flows through and connects everyone and everything in the universe. Ayurveda sees life as that exchange of energy and information between individuals and their extended body – the environment. If our environment is nourishing, we thrive; if our environment is toxic; we may become sick. Therefore, learning how to eliminate toxicity and surround ourselves with a healing environment is the key to good health.[4]

The spiritual significance of disease in Ayurveda is rooted in *karma* physical and mental illnesses are believed to be a suffering due to past bad karmas and karmic accounts accumulated in this life and from past lives.

Ayurvedas Holistic concepts of Health

Svasthya, is the ayurvedic term for health, however it is the state of optimal health. It is a state of equilibrium of the mind, body and spirit. In order to achieve this, one has to have a balance of many anatomic, physiologic, social and psychological factors. The key to good health or optimal health is energy balance of metabolic and excretory processes, body tissues balance, besides mental balance. In fact according to ayurvedic concept optimal health cannot be achieved unless one has attained a state of self-awareness and has to be in a state of contented self.[5]

Ten factors (*dasa vidha pariksa*) are used to determine the state of health of an individual per Ayurveda namely; state of body tissues (*dusya*), physical strength (*bala*), age (*vaya*), mental strength or temperament (*sattva*), habituation or how you live, state of hygiene (*satmya*), food (*ahara*) where you live (*desa*), seasons/time of the year (*kala*), digestive and metabolic processes (*agni or anala*), genetic constitution (*prakriti*) 6. All these factors are taken into consideration when the well-being or health of an individual is being assessed. While these are mainly used for diagnostic purposes, these can also be used to measure the wellbeing of an individual.

Ayurvedic Concept of the Doshas

According to Ayurveda there are five elements or *mahabhutas* that make up everything within our bodies and everything outside of our bodies: space, air, fire, water, and earth. Space carries all the aspects of pure potentiality – infinite possibilities, air has the qualities of movement and change, fire is hot, direct, and transformational, water is cohesive and protective, and earth is solid, grounded, and stable. [3]

Biological systems of the body intertwine these five forces into patterns known as *doshas*. They are most easily thought of as mind-body principles that govern our style of thinking and behaving. All three doshas are present in every cell, tissue, and organ. Most of us have one or two doshas, which are most lively in our nature.

The three doshas are known as *Vata, Pitta, & Kapha*

Vata dosha, woven from the elements of Space and Air, regulates movement and change in our minds and bodies. If we are predominantly Vata, we tend to be thin, light and quick in our thoughts and actions. Change is a constant part of our lives. When Vata is balanced, we are creative, enthusiastic and lively. But if Vata becomes excessive, we may develop anxiety, insomnia or irregular digestion.

Pitta dosha, comprises of Fire and Water, governs digestion and metabolism. If the Pitta dosha is most active in our nature, we tend to be muscular, smart and determined. If balanced, we are warm, intelligent and a good leader. If out of balance, Pitta can make us critical, irritable and aggressive.

Kapha dosha, made from Earth and Water. If we have mostly Kapha in our nature, we tend to have a heavier frame, think and move more leisurely and are stable, when balanced; it creates calmness, sweetness and loyalty. When excessive, Kapha can cause weight gain, congestion and resistance to healthy change.[4]

It is common for people to have a blend of characteristics and usually one will tend to be dominate

Using the principles of Ayurveda, we can identify our mind/body nature and use this understanding to make the most nourishing choices in our lives.

An important goal of Ayurveda is to identify a person's ideal state of balance, determine when they are out of balance, and offer interventions using diet, exercise (*yoga*) herbs, aromatherapy, massage treatments, music, and meditation to reestablish balance.

Knowing what your dosha is provides invaluable information that will help you get in touch with your body's inner intelligence.

Prakriti – A Guide to Personalize Diets and Scientific genomic correlations

An individual's *prakriti* is another important determinant of the effect of food on the system. Prakriti of an individual is characterized by a set of physical, physiological, and psychological attributes. For example, based on taste preference, individuals can be grouped as vata (having affinity for sweet, sour, and salty tastes); pitta (with liking for sweet, bitter, and astringent taste), and kapha (for pungent, bitter, and astringent tastes). Whereas these tastes mitigate any negative effects of the inherited constitution, usage of tastes in the reverse order can cause imbalance in the body. For example, if a vata constitution person continuously consumes pungent, bitter, and astringent tasting materials, it could lead to rapid aging and degeneration of the body [3,7.] It is interesting to note that the concept of personalized medicine, which is the future of medicine, has been practiced since thousands of years the difference is now laboratory analysis guide treatment decisions, but back the systematic observation, clinical characteristics and health outcomes guided personalized medicine.

According to Ayurveda, *prakriti* of a person is determined at the time of conception and does not change until death. Recommendations on diets, lifestyles, and drugs vary depending on the *prakriti* of the individual 3 Since it gets determined at the time of conception, the hypothesis that *prakriti* has a genetic basis was tested by different groups of Indian scientists. A correlation between specific *prakriti* and HLA-DRB1 polymorphism was demonstrated by Bhushan et al., 8 Prasher et al. 9 and Mukherjee and Prasher 10 have used *prakriti*-based classification and have demonstrated the genomic and biochemical correlates with specific *prakriti* types. They have termed this approach of classification of humans as *Ayurgenomics* and propose its potential use in personalized and preventive medicine. Frequency of association of CYP2C19 genotype was demonstrated to vary depending on the *prakriti* 11 Differential expression of a high-altitude adaptation gene, *EGLN1* as a response to hypoxia, was correlated to specific *prakriti* type[12]. Rotti et al.[13] found a significant correlation between dominant *prakriti* to place of birth and body mass index (BMI).

In contrast with conventional medicine, which has devoted a lot of effort to isolating the differences among various diseases, Ayurveda focuses on the unique qualities of individuals, pointing out that diseases differ mainly because people are so different. It is a more personalized form of management.

The Ayurvedic perspective on health and illness is the interconnection of all things. We aren't simply an isolated collection of atoms and molecules, but are an inseparable part of the infinite field of intelligence. From this holistic perspective, health isn't merely the absence of illness or symptoms - it is a higher state of consciousness that allows vitality, well-being, creativity, and joy to flow into our experience. In contrast, illness is a disruption - a blockage in the flow of energy and information that creates a sense of separation or alienation from the field. Symptoms and sickness are the body's signal that we need to restore balance, eliminate whatever is causing the blockages, and reestablish the healthy flow of energy and information.

Ayurveda teaches that all healing measures —dietary plan or herbal supplement or an exercise program, — must be based on an understanding of an individual's unique mind-body constitution or *dosha*. By knowing a patient's dosha, an Ayurvedic doctor can tell which diet, physical activities, and herbal therapies are most likely to help.

Ayurveda teaches that the mind has the greatest influence in directing the body toward sickness and health. Thousands of years before modern medicine "discovered" the mind-body connection, the ancient sages had mastered it. They developed Ayurveda as a system for contacting our own inner intelligence (or mind), bringing it into balance, and then extending that balance to the body.

Western medicine focuses on symptoms of disease; Ayurveda seeks to eliminate illness by treating the underlying cause. For example, for a patient suffering from depression, an allopathic physician would likely prescribe a standard course of antidepressants and, perhaps, therapy. An Ayurvedic doctor, on the other hand, would seek to understand the root imbalances contributing to the depression. The doctor would look at the patient as a whole, taking into consideration his or lifestyle, activities, diet, recent stressful events, beliefs, and mind-body constitution. The Ayurvedic practitioner would then recommend a healing holistic plan taking all of these factors into account.

Ahara (Food) a Pillar of Life

Ahara is one of the three pillars of life according to Ayurveda; the other two being sleep and regulated sexual life.

An interesting concept of Food is; Food is prescribed as per the body type dosha. Also food is classified on the effect it has on various body organs and also based on their impact on psychological constitution of an individual.

The classical texts of Ayurveda of 300 BC–700 AD dedicate elaborate sections on foods. 6 They describe the unique aspects including detailed descriptions of food and beverage. Food classification is based on food safety, taste, therapeutic qualities, etc. Different incompatibilities of food based on their tastes, processing, dose, time, and place also is considered during classification. The prescriptions of food consumption, food qualities and intake are based on the digestive ability of an individual, and the nature of food that is being consumed[3].

Taste (Rasa) as an Indicator of Health Effects

One of the ways of food classification in Ayurveda is based on is *rasa*. There are six major tastes according to Ayurveda, viz., sweet, sour, salty, pungent, bitter, and astringent. There are primary and secondary qualities (*guna*) that increase the properties of a material. This is further augmented by potency (*virya*), post-digestive effect (*vipaka*), and therapeutic action (*karma*). According to Ayurveda, the classification based on rasa, guna, virya, vipaka, and karma is not only applicable to foods but also for all materials, including medicines, and is dealt with under *Dravya guna sastra* (the science of materials' properties), the Ayurvedic pharmacology [14]

Food Can Alter Moods

According to Ayurveda, psychological states are closely linked to foods; there is a subtle link between disease manifestation and the six psychological expressions, such as lust, anger, greed, desire, attachment, and ego. This connection is further discussed in terms of three states of being including *sattva, rajas,* and *tamas*. Sattva is the contented state, rajas an excited state whereas tamas relates to a lethargic disposition, i.e., foods can induce these states of mind [15,16]

All this wisdom goes back to "you are what you eat" In ancient India food consumption was based of professional occupation and status in society. e.g the priests consumed pure vegetarian food or sattvic food which was devoid of excitation, the royals enjoyed rajas food rich in fat , including animal protein, nuts spices this type of food excited the senses. The tamas food was the stale food with low energy was provided to the working class.

Proper Metabolism is Key to Good Health

The energy that is derived by metabolic processes in the body was called *agni*, this is believed to have an important effect on health.

Incompatible Foods (Viruddha Ahara) and Processes

Yet another distinctive feature of Ayurveda is its understanding of incompatibilities of food materials and processing. There are 18 forms of incompatibilities according to Ayurveda [3]. Ayurveda eating according to the body type is a well-practiced art. There are many complex eating plans based on the body type, food is mostly plant based with inclusion of dairy form the local cows a different breed from the present day cows. Details are beyond scope of this book.

Wholesome and Unwholesome Food (Pathya and Apathya)

Several examples are provided in Ayurvedic texts in terms of wholesome supplements, *pathya* and *apathya*. These are particularly indicated in disease management. For example, pomegranate, amla (Indian gooseberry), buttermilk, etc. are mentioned as good *pathya ahara*. There are specific instructions to consume yogurt; that it should not be taken at night, or in seasons such as spring, summer, and fall. It should be taken with sugar cane candy (*gur*) or green gram soup or honey. There are also disease-specific or medicine-specific instructions that should be followed for consumption of food. As an example, a patient suffering from cough is advised to consume vegetables, such as coccinea; spices such as garlic and cardamom, long pepper, ginger, and condiments .It is also indicated that certain tastes have direct correlation with disease manifestation, hence, they are avoided during treatment of those conditions. There are also detailed descriptions of convalescence foods too.

From the above section, it is clear that Ayurveda has its own universally applicable principles, methods, and practices that are very different from biomedicine and modern nutrition concepts. Several efforts are ongoing to understand and interpret Ayurveda. A recurring criticism has been that natural science research in Ayurveda has been not adequately effective and has been limited to ethnobotany, biochemistry, and pharmacology. Most research initiatives till last few years were restricted to looking for compounds or molecules from Ayurveda drugs that could be absorbed to the modern pharmacopeia. These have not resulted in any substantial contributions in terms of new diagnostic techniques, formulations, or treatment approaches in Ayurveda except for some minor outcomes of validating certain Ayurvedic practices. This illustrates a distinct need to focus on fundamental research based on Ayurvedic principles for identifying new pathways and for more holistic perspectives in preventive as well as curative healthcare. There is much to be researched into the unique Ayurvedic concepts in nutrition, including *pathya, viruddha ahara, kala* and *desa vicara, agni, ama*, etc.

Mindful eating and Ayurveda

Upayoga samstha is the Ayurvedic term for mindful eating. It is a guideline for how to eat mindfully. The philosophy *Upayoga samstha* recommends

- Ayurveda emphasizes freshly cooked food consumed within half hour of cooking, as stale food loses its *prana* (life force)

- Eat warm food as cold food reduces *Agni* and the power of digestion

- Eat the right quantity of food. The person based on body type, levels of activity, should decide this. It is recommended to fill our stomach half with food, one quarter with water and one quarter with air.

- Giving full attention to the food you eat. It advises chewing the food thoroughly; eating at a moderate pace, enjoying the sight, smell, taste and texture of the food.

- Stop eating when satisfied. Eating the right quantity of food is emphasized.

- Eat only when hungry as hunger stimulates agni and digestive fire. Eating without hunger can lead to indigestion and heavy feeling.

- Ayurveda emphasizes a meal time routine when food is consumed in a regular time the body knows when to expect food and in anticipation it secretes digestive enzymes to support the physiological function of digestion.

- Have a regular gap between meals three hours is recommended. Constantly and haphazardly snacking can lead to digestive imbalances.

- It was recommended to eat in a peaceful surrounding. Food was considered an energy source so unsettled environment can enguf one in negative energy. In this situation one is likely to overeat, eat more quickly and then suffer from digestive issues.

- If one is upset one should not eat. One should wait till emotions are calmed down. Ayurveda believes if food is consumed with a disturbed mind it can be toxic to the body.

- Always sit down to eat. Actually in Ancient times it was recommended to sit on the floor in *padamasana* pose to eat food. Food had to be honored a small prayer was commenced before consuming the food.

- After the meal it was recommended to sit in *vajraasana* to help in digestion

Rasayana

Rasayana is a branch of Ayurveda that deals with means to enhance quality of life and extend lifespan. *Rasayana*s are useful in preventive, promotive, and curative health. They are said to mainly act in three possible ways (i) *Agnivyapara*: by regulating *agni* that drives transformations in the body, like the metabolic processes, (ii) *Srotosodhana*: by clearing the macro and micro channels thereby increasing tissue perfusion, and (iii) *Posana*: by nourishing tissues

- It mentions plants, animal products, metals, and minerals that can be used as *Rasayana* materials to delay aging and enhance wellbeing.

- Yoga is an integral part of Ayurveda in general and is a Rasayana

- It also describes the non-material-based methods, including meditation, good thoughts, conduct, and lifestyle that can influence well-being.

- Apart from tissue nourishment or perfusion, it is also to create balance of *dosa*

- Fasting is an important Rasayana for body healing.

- With the aging population growing these days *Rasayana* is a subject of research interest as focus is on anti-aging, rejuvenation, and wellness. Age-related diseases, such as Alzheimer's, Parkinson's, arthritis, atherosclerosis, and so on, can benefit by scientific research on the concept of *Rasayana*.

- Contemporary bioassay tools such as *in vitro* and small organisms such as Drosophila, *Caenorhabditis elegans*, yeast are now being used to observe the physical, physiological, and behavioral effect of *Rasayana*s and gain insights into the molecular mechanisms of action [17] Several studies have shown that *Rasayana* plants have anti-oxidant, adaptogenic [18]_anti-inflammatory[19-21] , anti-cancer [2] and anthelmintic [23] activities.

- *Medhya Rasayana* (Ayurvedic nootropics) such as Ashvagandha, turmeric, and brahmi have demonstrated the ability to clear amyloid-β plaques in neurons that are observed in Alzheimer's disease [24.] Research into *Rasayana* holds the potential to unravel diet and herbs-based preventive methods to curb neurodegeneration and aging, in general.

Ayurveda and of wisdom of fasting

Keeping a fast is an integral part of the Indian culture and all traditional Indian religions; Hindu, Christains, Bhudhist, Jains and Muslim live a lifestyle of regular fasting culture and this has been so for last thousands of years. Hindus call fasting "vrat' one willingly abstains from certain kind of food. The fast can range from half a day to up to 40 days or even more. There are mentions about fasting in many ancient Indian religious scriptures. As per most Hindu sacred books like the Bhagwad Gita and others, fasting helps create a connection with the Absolute by establishing a harmonious relationship between the body and the soul. Fasting is believed to be a great instrument for inculcating self-discipline. People fasted for many reasons they believe it is a kind of penance for sins and believed fasting can purify the soul. Most also believe fasting is the best detoxification tool.

However we would like to mention some key points; Ayurveda recommends fasting, as it believes it can initiate a number of metabolic adjustments and initiate powerful healing. Most of the herbal healing recipes in chapter7 are rooted in this ancient healing science based on centuries of observation.

Modern science is slowly discovering the benefits of fasting

- Fasting leads to longevity by stimulating autophagy and improving overall health.

- Fasting is a powerful detoxification tool; can reduce oxidative stress to the body, decrease inflammation, and protect from cancers

- Fasting can be used as a natural reset for the body especially if the body is exposed to excesses in food, toxins, or the environment.

- Fasting can help many in their attempts at balancing weight the health benefits include; reduced risk of diabetes, balancing lipid profile, reducing cardiovascular risk, improve blood pressure.

- Intermittent fasting kicks off a set of processes in the body, as the release of more *Norepinephrine,* an organic chemical in the catecholamine family that functions in the brain and body as a hormone and neurotransmitter, giving the person practicing the fast more energy, alertness, and focus. This leads to mental sharpness and creativity.

Water, Herbs and spices can support fasting so that it becomes easy for people to sail through the fasting window.

During the "eating window "people can eat according to their ayurveda body type for a better impact on health. Alternatively they can consume more vegetables and plant based food for a greater impact on health.

Interestingly the Ayurvedic practitioners by keen observation over period of thousand years discovered insulin resistance, eating according to neutrogenomic profile, and also Autophagy.

Some Ayurvedic fasting strategies

Spring is the "kapha" season and intense fasting is advised during this season if we associate with nature fall is season of abundance and by spring in ancient time's food stores would have been depleted so fasting was logical. Another logic for this fasting is any body fat stores accumulated in winter season could be balanced by the fasting.

Ayurveda recommends once a week fasting, it also recommends regular cleanses as it is believed that some food is toxic to the body systems and fasting is the antidote for this. Various fasting regimes have been suggested Medicinal Herbs and Spices formed a very vitally important support for fasting.

Liquid fast: This is said to balance the fire component in the body. Liquid days involve drinking liquids and herbal concoctions (refer to recipe section). On these days a liquid vegetable soup is prepared and you can consume this along with herbal teas practically every 2 hours. The fast gives the system a chance to heal and rejuvenate. Ayurvedic liquid fasting can be incorporated in life once a week so that you can reap the benefits to your health.

On the next day a light "Khichdi "is recommended (recipe in recipe section) this has many medicinal herbs and spices to balance metabolism.

Ayurveda has a number of advanced therapeutic cleansing protocols described as "Kriyas "e.g. breath control, water therapy, colonic washes, ingestion of ghee a form of fat fast etc.

The Vedic Mono-diet Cleanse

One-Way to think of food is as information for the body. Actually, it really is the science of neutrogenomics is based on this fact. Food, like all matter, is comprised of atomic particles organized in a particular pattern. When we eat we take these in, break them down with enzymes, and reassemble them into new cellular structures. In the mono-cleanse diet only one type of food is ingested. Now with neutrogenomic science all these facts are being rediscovered. The ancient practitioners used this tool to exclude food and correlated the effects on healing.

The Ayurvedic principles for restoring and maintaining mind-body balance are as relevant today as they were thousands of years ago The least you can do based on Ayurvedic principles is:

1. Take time each day to quiet your mind Increase your spiritual Intelligence. (Meditate, Gratitude's and prayers).
2. Enjoy a clean diet comprising of fresh food according to your dosas; eat a colorful, flavorful diet. Eat plant-based diet.
3. Eat mindfully
4. Regularly have probiotics with meals.
5. Engage in Yoga or daily exercise that enhances flexibility, strength, and cardiovascular fitness.
6. Sleep soundly at night.
7. Eliminate what is not serving you; manage stress, Declutter, Detoxify your environment.
8. Cultivate loving, nurturing relationships. Learn tolerance and forgiveness
9. Perform your good Karma work that awakens your passion, gives purpose and meaning to your life and be happy

References

1. Sharma PV, editor. *History of Medicine in India*. New Delhi: Indian National Science Academy (1992). p. vii–xii.
2. Anonymous. *Report of Procedings: International Workshop-Integrating Traditional South-Asian Medicine into Modern Healthcare Systems*. New Delhi: Jawaharlal Nehru University (2015).
3. Sharma PV, editor. *Caraka Samhita*. (Vol. 1). Varanasi: Chaukhambha Orientalia (2001). p. 5–9,190,228,375–6.
4. Sharma PV, editor. *Susrutha Samhitha*. (Vol. 1). Varanasi: Chaukhambha Visvabharati (2004). 173 p.
5. Payyappallimana U, Venkatasubramanian P. In: Verotta L, Pia Macchi M, Venkatasubramanian P, editors. *Principles of Ayurveda for Food, Nutrition,*

and Health in Connecting Indian Wisdom and Western Science – Plant Usage for Nutrition and Health. New York: CRC Press (2015). p. 15–36.

6. Murthy KRS, editor. *Vagbhata's Astanga Hrdayam.* 5th ed. (Vol. **1**). Varanasi: Chaukhambha Orientalia (2001). p. 53–7.

7. Dey S, Pahwa P. *Prakriti* and its associations with metabolism, chronic diseases, and genotypes: possibilities of new born screening and a lifetime of personalized prevention. *J Ayurveda Integr Med* (2014) **5**(1):15–24. doi:10.4103/0975-9476.128848

8. Bhushan P, Kalpana J, Arvind C. Classification of human population based on HLA gene polymorphism and the concept of Prakriti in Ayurveda. *J Altern Complement Med* (2005) **11**(2):349–53.

9. Prasher B, Negi S, Aggarwal S, Mandal AK, Sethi TP, Deshmukh SR, et al. Whole genome expression and biochemical correlates of extreme constitutional types defined in ayurveda. *J Transl Med* (2008) **6**:48. doi:10.1186/1479-5876-6-48

10. Mukerji M, Prasher B. Ayurgenomics: a new approach in personalized and preventive medicine. *Sci Cult.* New Delhi, India: Institute of Genomics and Integrative Biology (2011) **77**(1–2):10–7.

11. Ghodke Y, Joshi K, Patwardhan B. Traditional medicine to modern pharmacogenomics: ayurveda prakriti type and CYP2C19 gene polymorphism associated with the metabolic variability. *Evid Based Complement Alternat Med* (2011) **2011**:249528. doi:10.1093/ecam/nep206

12. Aggarwal S, Negi S, Jha P, Singh PK, Stobdan T, Pasha MA, et al. EGLN1 involvement in high-altitude adaptation revealed through genetic analysis of extreme constitution types defined in ayurveda. *Proc Natl Acad Sci U S A* (2010) **107**(44):18961–6. doi:10.1073/pnas.1006108107

13. Rotti H, Raval R, Anchan S, Bellampalli R, Bhale S, Bharadwaj R, et al. Determinants of prakriti, the human constitution types of Indian traditional medicine and its correlation with contemporary science. *J Ayurveda Integr Med* (2014) **5**(3):167–75. doi:10.4103/0975-9476.140478

14. Dhyani SC. *Rasapanchaka.* Varanasi: Krishnadas Academy (1994). p. 32–42, 46–60.

15. Prabhupada BS, editor. *Bhagavadgita Yatharupa.* 19th ed. Bangalore: ISKCON (2002). p. 736–8. [Kannada Language translation].

16. Murthy KRS, editor. *Astanga Samgraha of Vagbhata.* 1st ed. (Vol. **2**). Varanasi: Chaukhambha Orientalia (1996). 102 p.

17. Dwivedi V, Anandan EM, Mony RS, Muraleedharan TS, Valiathan MS, Mutsuddi M, et al. In vivo effects of traditional ayurvedic formulations

in *Drosophila melanogaster* model relate with therapeutic applications. *PLoS One* (2012) **7**(5):e37113. doi:10.1371/journal.pone.0037113

18. Rege NN, Thatte UM, Dahanukar SA. Adaptogenic properties of six rasayana herbs used in ayurvedic medicine. *Phytother Res* (1999) **13**(4):275–91. doi:10.1002/(SICI)1099-1573.

19. Shyni GL, Ratheesh M, Sindhu G, Helen A. Anti-inflammatory and antioxidant effects of Jeevaneeya Rasayana: an ayurvedic polyherbal formulation on acute and chronic models of inflammation. *Immunopharmacol Immunotoxicol* (2010) **32**(4):569–75. doi:10.3109/08923970903584890

20. Aggarwal BB, Prasad S, Reuter S, Kannappan R, Yadev VR, Park B, et al. Identification of novel anti-inflammatory agents from ayurvedic medicine for prevention of chronic diseases: "reverse pharmacology" and "bedside to bench" approach. *Curr Drug Targets* (2011) **12**(11):1595–653.

21. Singh AK. Rationality of rasayana therapy as adoptogenic, antioxidant and anti-inflammatory agent. *Intl Res J Pharm* (2011) **2**(12):259–60.

22. Datta S, Mishra RN. *Plumbago zeylinica* Linn. (Chitrak) – review as rasayan (rejuvenator/antiaging). *Int J Res Pharm Biomed Sci* (2012) **3**(1):250–6

23. Venkatasubramanian P, Godbole A, Vidyashankar R, Kuruvilla GR. Evaluation of traditional anthelmintic herbs as substitutes for the endangered *Embelia ribes*, using *Caenorhabditis elegans* model. *Curr Sci* (2013) **105**(11):1593–8.

24. Tiwari SK, Pandey YK. Ayurvedic drugs in prevention and management of age related cognitive decline: a review. *Int J Pharm Sci Drug Res* (2012) **4**(3):183–90.

CHAPTER 5
FROM KNOWLEDGE AND WISDOM TO ACTION

At the individual level "Swaraj" is connected with the capacity for dispassionate self-assessment, ceaseless self –purification and growing self-reliance. It is Swaraj when we learn to rule ourselves.
-Mahatma Gandhi, Young India, 28th June 1928

Swaraj means ruling over ourselves. In the present context it is so important that we realize the importance of Swaraj as this is the biggest power we have when it comes to nutrition.

As mentioned earlier we now know how addicting the chemical combination of natural food substances like all the sugar and sugar like substances can be. The man-made chemicals like MSG besides being addicting are even toxic.

To broadly simplify the action plan and to make the messages easy to remember we have classified the actions in Five R s Remove, Replace, Restore, Retrain and Rehabilitate.

Remove

The Great pantry purge

Hope you are ready for the action as it's going to be hard to say goodbye to your food friends: the bags of chips, cookies chocolates. Many will be easy to spot few will be mischievously hiding and masquerading as aliases. Just we need to remember they are taking more from us than they are giving us back. Just ask yourself whether the food item is contributing or interfering with your goal of achieving optimal health.

Start the process early on when you are in a fully motivational state. Get a large bag and start purging from the fridge, freezer and pantry. What you do with the food is your preference- donate to a local food bank, donation center, friends and family. You may be tempted to hide the stuff thinking "out of sight out of mind "somewhere for later use, however be aware that strong will power is a rare thing, you definitely don't want to slip during a weak emotional moment then blame yourself later for emotional eating.

For people with kids and families –just remember you are doing your family a huge service by this heath-protecting act. It's amazing how many children improve their focus, mental and spiritual wellbeing by following this new way of eating.

1. Remove all boxed **processed** food with a long list of ingredients.
2. Dump **Sugar and its relatives** anything with ose at the end or syrup: high fructose corn syrup, and the sugar substitutes. Sugars substitutes are also very detrimental to health as firstly they can contribute to insulin resistance and they are toxic to the microbiome. Some more reasons for dumping sugar are: Sugar is an addictive drug. Research has shown that it is worse than cocaine. When consumed it causes a dopamine rush in the brain stimulating pleasure, when withdrawn it can cause opiate like withdrawal symptoms depression and anxiety. It can cause craving. Sure we all have experienced having a bite of a sweet treat leads to another and then we can't stop. Sugar can cause insulin resistance –This can lead to metabolic syndrome, cardiovascular disease, type 2 diabetes and obesity. It can cause cancer as cancer is closely

related to elevated insulin levels. Sugar is also known to cause vitamin and mineral deficiencies. Finally research has shown that Sugar can shorten your life span –Research has shown regular sugar consumers have shorter telomeres this is an indication of accelerated DNA degeneration and aging. So dump the sugar and its relatives.

3. Remove **wheat and all gluten** containing food: The major reason for avoiding gluten is that 30-50% of populations are sensitive to gluten. Most go undiagnosed if you suffer from digestive problems, headaches, eczemas, fatigue, and brain fog try avoiding the gluten. Gluten is hiding in a whole lot of processed food- baked goodies, pastas, soy sauce, most seasonings, stuffing's, cereal bars, stock cubes, hydrolyzed proteins and malt vinegar. Most of us have experienced visiting restaurants and devouring the bread from the breadbasket to our surprise and dismay. It's not our fault, wheat is addicting a protein called Gliadin when digested becomes an exorphin an morphine like compound that stimulate opiate receptors in the brain. Wheat also has phytic acid, oxalic acid and lectins in a later section we discuss this in detail. Wheat also has amylopectin A, which is responsible for expansion of visceral fat causing "wheat belly". It also causes sugar spikes and insulin spikes. Lectin and gluten together cause a condition known as "leaky gut "this can cause a storm for the immune system and result in serious auto –immune disorders.

4. Get rid of **the GMO** soy; it has phytic acid, oxalic acid and lectins. Soy is hiding in most Asian food, processed food, protein bars, protein powders vegetable burgers , Mayonnaise, and vegetable oil.

5. Hunt and get rid of **Monosodium glutamate and its aliases**. Refer page 17 for detains on MSG.

6. Get rid of **plastics**; never microwave in plastic containers, get rid of plastic containers, use glass jars and containers, wrap your food in paper rather than plastic.

7. Take care of the **phytates** –As you start a plant based diet your exposure to Phytates increases they are present in beans seeds chia seed flax seed, nuts cereal grains, brown rice and oats. One way of dealing with this is soaking, washing, sprouting and fermenting these grains and seeds.

8. **Oxalates** – fount in raw spinach, wheat buckwheat, peanuts, beans, sweet potatoes, quinoa, nuts, celery potatoes, okra, tomatoes and carrots. Oxalates can cause kidney stones and interfere with vitamin and mineral absorption. Boiling reduces oxalates .Raw vegans need to take care of oxalates

9. **Lectins**- Lectins can make us fat as they attach to insulin receptors in fat cells once they latch on they never detach, they also attach themselves to receptor sites for leptin, the satiety hormone. Lectin also contribute to leaky gut. Foods high in lectin are brown rice, wheat, spelt, rye, barley, soy beans, beans, seeds, nuts, corn, potato skin, eggplant and all peppers. Heat destroys lectin especially pressure-cooking. Soaking beans with frequent water changing can remove the lectin.

10. **Trypsin inhibitors** – They are found in soybeans, grains, nuts, seeds, nightshade vegetables – potatoes, tomatoes and eggplants. These are plants natural pest repellant, they cause havoc with digestion, and prevent vitamin and mineral absorption. Trypsin inhibitors add stress to the pancreas leading to pancreatitis, and even pancreatic cancer. Luckily cooking destroys the trypsin inhibitors. Raw vegans need to take care of the risks from Trypsin inhibitors.

11. **Phosphoric acid**: it is found in bubbly drinks and flavored water. Phosphoric acid leaches bone of calcium disturbs digestion, disturbs vitamin and mineral uptake by the body.
12. Lastly but not the least; Remove the non-organic, antibiotic laden, hormone laden **animal protein** food; dairy, eggs, poultry, and meats.

Replace

The Ancient wisdom food that stays

1. Replace the above food with the foods that are natural, unprocessed or minimally processed "Plant based Whole food" These are high in nutrients, your grandmother used them. They provide you nourishment and are compatible with your personalized eating plan. The Organic vegetables, Non- GMO vegetables, and fruit stay. Since you'll be eating mostly Plant based. Replace processed food by Vegetables, which are probably the most nutrient dense food group in terms of macronutrients and micronutrients. They are low in calories but high in vitamins, minerals and fiber. Low carbohydrate vegetables do not spike blood sugar. Cruciferous vegetables like cauliflower, broccoli, cabbage, Brussels sprouts are rich in glucosinolates which prevent cancer, slow tumor growth, and reduce inflammation. By choosing a diet rich in vegetables you will feel an overall sense of wellbeing and increased energy. By adopting a diet rich in vegetables you may be able to significantly reduce the risk of developing type2 diabetes, heart disease, stroke and cancer.
2. Frozen Vegetables are mildly processed they stay as the convenience of having frozen vegetables is huge more over frozen veges have been picked at the right time so the nutrient content is good at times even better than stale store bought fresh vegetables.

3. Replace wheat, soy with Gluten free ancient grains like, buckwheat, Amaranth, Shorgum rice, Millets , Fox tail millet , Quinoa .

4. Replace dairy with nut milk incorporate seeds like flax seed, chia seed and other seeds. Replace peanuts with almond nut, walnut, pecans. Ancient grains and seeds are all excellent Low carb high fiber foods.

5. Since we are going mostly plant based instead of animal protein add sources of plant protein there are so many lentils that can be chosen, pea protein, beans quinoa are a good source of amino-acids One of the best sources of plant protein is hemp seeds.

6. To minimize the toxins in grains and seeds, wash, rinse, Sprout and pressure-cook beans.

7. The most difficult but also most rewarding is replacing sugar with whole fruit, whole fruit has fiber, and this prevents sugar rushes. If weight loss is a goal you can stick to low glycemic fruit like berries, peaches, papaya and apples. Still we need to remember fruit is not a free food can be had in limited quantities only.

8. Use fresh herbs and spices to make food more flavorful.

9. Don't compromise on taste replace all food with MSG and its aliases with homemade seasonings.

10. If you need to consume meat :Replace store bought factory farmed meat and poultry with organically farm raised cage free poultry, wild caught fish and grass fed meat. Try to consume very small or tiny amounts of animal protein from free range, organic antibiotic hormone free poultry and eggs, grass fed lamb, beef or even wild meat.

Try to buy locally, try to buy seasonally, support your local farmers. Even if you need to pay a bit more, at least you know the source of the food, more over since you will be saving by not buying processed food and minimizing eating out in the long run you will not be spending a lot.

Restore

Revamp

Microbiome

1. The first step to revamp your microbiome is to increase your plant-based food there are many reasons for this firstly the plants have fiber and this insoluble fiber goes to the colon and helps the beneficial bacteria multiply. Raw vegetables are a rich source of bacteria.

2. If your diet has a lot of diversity or vegetables, more different kind of bacteria get their nutrition and it is like a fertilizer for the microbiome research has also shown that in case there is less vegetable plant fiber in the colon the bacteria eat the gut lining and this can contribute to leaky gut if there is an abundance of good bacteria that nourish the intestinal cells with Short Chain Fatty Acids and heal the leaky gut.

3. Go fermented to include these friendly bacteria as a daily health food.

    One of the biggest secrets for developing a very healthy microbiome is to increase the consumption of fermented foods the fermented foods are not only in friendly bacteria but also contain the fiber which is important for them to multiply the ancient wisdom has shown that eating fermented food with every meal can really help your microbiome in the long run so it's better to develop a lifestyle habit of including fermented food and every meal the end of the book has recipes to delicious fermented food

4. Prebiotics are fermentable compounds that help friendly bacteria grow and thrive. While probiotic foods contain live bacteria, prebiotic foods boost the good bacteria by feeding the good

bacteria already living in the digestive system. Prebiotics are present in foods such as asparagus, artichokes, bananas, oatmeal, red wine, honey, maple syrup, and legumes.

To boost friendly bacteria in the intestines, include prebiotics in your diet (fiber rich foods that contain non digestible carbohydrates, e.g., oatmeal, flaxseed, onions, garlic, leeks, asparagus, chicory roots).

Try to increase your intake of prebiotic food like resistant starch and inulin some food which are high in resistant starch include green bananas green banana flour, green peas, white beans lentils and uncooked rolled oats these resistant starch a very important because they feed the bacteria the in the gut. It is found in leeks, garlic, and onions so by adding them to your vegetables not only will improve the taste of the food you eat but will also help your microbiome

5. If you want reduce your milk and meat intake as these are not good for the microbial because meat might be raised with hormones and antibiotics besides that research has shown the L-Carnitine in red meat and animal protein can get converted to a chemical trimethylamine –N-oxide (TMAO) this has been associated with artery clogging plaque formation so you increase the chances of heart attacks and stroke it is better to avoid meat completely but if you cannot then you can reduce the milk and meat consumption and try to have grass fed meat and organically raised poultry try to be very careful about the animal protein you consume by carefully studying the source and labels.

6. Avoid sugar as much as you can studies have shown that sugar consumption leads to overgrowth of yeast and other bad bacteria this leads to increased craving for sugar you can gradually reduce the consumption of sugar and slowly your gut bacteria will alter and they no longer crave sugar. Artificial sweeteners are equally

bad as they have been shown to lead to glucose intolerance and which is a major factor for developing diabetes.

7. Avoiding processed food is also recommended, as it is believed that good bacteria don't like preservatives and other harsh chemicals. Besides chemicals and hormones most of these food have the fiber stripped from them so this is all not good for the GI tract avoid food like gluten refined carbohydrates dairy processed foods in general GMO fruits and foods with artificial sweeteners all these have shown to destroy the friendly gut bacteria.

8. Watch out for things and situations that will disrupt good versus bad microbes. Like taking antibiotics as these indiscriminately kill all microbes and lead to overgrowth of unfriendly microbes and yeast fungi like Candida.

9. Other unfriendly and health enemies that disrupt this balance are H-pylori, periodontal disease, vaginal infections, upper respiratory tract infections, urinary tract infections, and fungal skin infections.

10. Choosing a probiotic supplement is a difficult task. One really needs to do their homework; the average probiotic dose of yoghurt is too low, according to experts. Different strains have different benefits. For example, vaginal yeast responds to *lactobacillus rhamnosus GR1* and *lactobacillus reuteri RC14*. Supplements need to be stored properly, and often need to be refrigerated as the bacterial colonies drop with time and with storage at unsuitable temperatures.

Caution: People who have a suppressed immune system or those on chemotherapy need to be cautious with these bacterial foods.

Retrain

1. Retrain yourselves and your family for a lifestyle change incorporating the new Canada food guidelines. Even if one can

stick to the new guidelines 80% of the time a big impact can be noticed in health.

2. Educate yourself in nutrition read books, use web information, and attend seminars. In the long run this might turn out to be one of the best retraining you have undertaken for your mind body and spirit.

3. Gradually retrain your taste buds to accept healthy options in food like vegetables and especially bitter tasting green vegetables instead of sweet desserts

4. Eat home cooked meals, encourage all, family community to cook at home. The benefits to health by this one retraining is going to change so much for every one; you will know what has gone into the food, toxins can be completely eliminated. With time your food enjoyment will surge

5. Learn how to ferment food and prepare probiotics at home, so that they can be had with every meal. Refer to recipe section.

6. Learn to cook international cuisines like Middle eastern, Japanese, Chinese, Indian, Thai, Malaysian these cuisines are very much plant based as unlike North America and other prosperous countries these communities could never afford large amounts of animal protein, so the food from these continents contains only small amounts of animal protein. However remember to use high quality ingredients only.

7. Practice mindful eating refer chapter on Ayurveda for retraining in mindful eating

Rehabilitate

1. We need to recognize that food has been a major addiction to many of us. This fact has been kept under wraps by the food politics, food industries, and media. If everyone wakes up to these facts who is going to grease the wheels of capitalism. So communities, individuals and countries need to wake up and return people to good health by rehabilitation at every level. Considerable effort

from individuals, society, communities and countries is needed. Canada has taken a first step by keeping its people's health interest as a priority in spite of pressures from the industry

2. Inactivity has taken epidemic proportions so there needs to be a huge rehabilitation program to get populations to Exercise more. You can take an initiative and exercise at least half hour walk every day.

3. Sleep hygiene is another big unrecognized menace for which people need to be rehabilitated.

4. Stress management needs to be focused on.

5. Local rehabilitation programs under motivated leadership of communities are needed.

6. At a personal level I can think of rehabilitation programs for people with severe addictions are available in India in the Ayurvedic farms where people check in for a month or more and are fully rejuvenated often free of many chronic illnesses and symptoms. There are also many nutritional rehabs around the US Mexico border. People checking into these rehabilitation centers have returned cured of cardiac conditions, some even needed surgery, and were spared from surgery. These programs even claim to cure diabetes, hypertension and many autoimmune conditions.

CHAPTER 6.
DEVELOPING A CUSTOMIZED ACTION PLAN

"Eat food, not too, much mostly plants"
Michael Pollan

Personalized Nutrition is what we aim to achieve.

Personalized Nutrition based on genomic typing and micro biome typing is the best action plan one can go for, unfortunately very few would have access to these advanced plans.

By now we all know Diet and nutrition interact, so we are predisposed for dietary susceptibility. Developing a personalized nutritional plan involves consideration of what your personal goals are, medical, family histories. By now we also know that what might be a great eating pattern for someone else might be unsuitable for another person. For those who have access to testing for biomarkers and genetic variants and those who can get a "nutritional blue print" can follow that path blending with their eater identity. There are challenges in following this type of eating as eating socially can be a huge challenge. Personalized nutrition is still in infancy and is an evolving trend.

Some of us can try vedic nutrition that is eating according to body type. However details of this type of eating is beyond scope of this book. It takes time but gradually people get used to eating in this patern. This too has its limitations as it is quite specific very labor intensive to prepare and may be challenging to get ingredients. The eating plan has big customized herbal supplement list.

Recognize the importance of mind game in relation to food. We cannot ignore the effect of negative and positive emotions on the body.

To summarize the Ancient Wisdom rules which everyone can apply in general:

The General 7 Ancient wisdom Rules for today's Food

Ancient Wisdom Rule 1

Eat Whole food plant based meals, try to eat local seasonal and clean organic. Try to focus on plant based protein If at all, eat a minimum occasional very small amount of clean animal protein (Organic free range, grass fed).

Ancient Wisdom Rule 2

Sack Sugar, Wheat and Soy and their aliases. Sack processed food with many ingredients.

Ancient Wisdom Rule 3

Eliminate the obesogens and their aliases: MSG,BPA, Phthalates and other Toxins- like Oxalates, Tannins, Phosphoric acid, reduce caffeine and Alcohol (no more than 2 servings per day).

Ancient Wisdom Rule 4

Eat probiotics and prebiotics with every meal hopefully some day we will have a research based daily requirement for probiotics. For this book I have come to the following estimation based on the doses used by scientists in published research.

1. If you are healthy try to consume at least 1-2 servings per day, 4 oz. yoghurt/ Kefir with label 'live and active cultures" is one serving, 1.5 oz. cheese is one serving. For people sensitive to dairy use coconut kefir.

2. If you are aiming to prevent medical problems consume 2-3 servings/day.
3. Select foods that contain a variety of probiotics (fermented foods, kimchi pickles, miso etc.)
4. Remember it is beneficial to have the probiotics with every meal, so space out supplementation over the day
5. People with diagnosed immune disorders can have commercial probiotic capsules even Human strain probiotics.
6. Given the fresh reports on poor purity of supplements and loss of colonies in commercial supplements due to storage, it is preferable to include probiotic food to one's routine diet as a conscious life style choice. Besides tasting great it is a wonder Health food.

Ancient Wisdom Rule 5

Supplement diet with micronutrients customized to your needs as follows:

1. For Young healthy Normal Females the prevention recommendations are One Multivitamin with minerals, Iron 18 mgm per day, need to take it separately not with other supplements. Vitamin D 1000 IU daily, Omega 3 – 2-3 helpings of fatty fish /week, 3 tbsp ground flax seed, Vitamin E, Magnesium 300 mgm /day Gama Lilonic Acid GLA –Evening primrose Oil, borage oil
2. For healthy Normal males the prevention recommendations are: One Multivitamin with minerals (check for calcium better to avoid), Vitamin D 1000 IU daily, Vitamin C 1000mgm/day, Zinc gluconate or piclinate 40 mgm daily, Magnesium 300 mgm /day ,Omega 3 – 2-3 helpings of fatty fish /week , 3 tbsp ground flax seed.
3. Supplements for Brain Health: Vitamins B complex are used during neurotransmission. Niacin B3 has been shown to improve memory. Vitamin supplementation has been recommended for

brain function. Vitamin E   2000/IU/day has shown to slow progression of AD, Riboflavin 200 mg ,Coenzyme 10 100-200 mg, Vitamin E 400-800 IU ,Essential oil formula, Magnesium , Calcium. Herbal supplements like turmeric and Ginkobiloba

4. Supplements for bone Health: This is a basic list for osteoporosis, arthritis and gout. Folic acid 20-60 mgm, Calcium 800mg-1 gm, Vitamin D 1000-4000iu, Vitamin C 1-3 gm , Magnesium 400-800 mgm, B-complex 50-100mg, Choindroitin sulfate 50-150 mg, Glucosamin 1000-2000mg, Essential oil formula 300-7,000mg, and Zinc 20-30 mgm

5. Anti aging: Of the various approaches to slow down the aging process, calorie restriction is considered the gold standard. At present the scientific community, the government, and even the news media are slowly recognizing that our concept of extending life is in fact technically feasible, there is suggestive scientific evidence that they significantly suppress damaging free radical and inflammatory reactions that are linked to underlying aging processes. Intermittent Fasting is invaluable refer to book on Intermittent fasting with herbs and spices. The anti Aging supplements include: **Astaxanthine,** Coenzyme Q10 , Acetyle-L-Carnitine, Arginate, Asprin , Carnosine, Fish oil, Green Tea Extract, Lipolic Acid, Resverartol, Whey protein, BComplex Vitamins- Folic Acid, Vitamin B6&VitaminB12.

6. Supplements for heart health: We suggest that when planning a supplement program for improving risk factors for heart disease you work with a nutritionally oriented physician who can help you decide which supplements and doses are best for you. If you take medications, this is particularly important because certain supplements can react with or magnify the effects of certain drugs.

Again we would like lay emphasis; supplements cannot replace good lifestyle habits of Diet, exercise, and emotional health.

For people who are at risk of heart disease- that practically includes anyone with the metabolic syndrome, prediabetes, or diabetes we recommend several **antioxidant** vitamins and minerals as well as some nutrients, Vitamin C 1, 000- 2000 mg/day, Vitamin E- 400-800 IU/Day, B Vitamins- Folic acid, Vitamin B3, Vitamin B6 and Vitamin B12, Magnesium, Taurine for high blood pressure, Omega 3 fatty acid, Coenzyme Q10.

7. Supplements for Blood Sugar Control, Insulin Resistance and Obesity Supplements have to supplement Healthy lifestyle; Low glycemic, low carbohydrate Diet, Aerobic and Anaerobic exercises, and Emotional balance. The list includes following optimum doses need to be determined with an Integrative medicine practitioner. Natural probiotic with every meal One Mineral Multivitamin supplement daily, Vitamin B group B3, B5, B6,B7, Vitamin D 1000 -2000 iu daily, Magnesium 200-800 mgm /day,Chromium 200-1000gm/day , L-Argenine 500-2000g/day.
Herbal supplements: Garlic 3 gm/day, bitter mellon, Psyllium 5-10 gms/day, Garcinia Gambogia, Ginseng, fenugreek etc there is a long list of herbal supplements for weight loss.

Ancient Wisdom Rule 6
Do not underestimate the power of exercise; the minimum is half hour per day or 7 thousand steps. Incorporation of YOGA can have a strong impact on overall health.

Ancient Wisdom Rule 7
Practice mindful eating as recommended by Ayurveda

- Give full attention to the food you eat; enjoy the sight, smell, taste and texture of the food.
- Chew the food thoroughly, eating at a moderate pace, stop eating when satisfied.
- Eat the right quantity of food.
- Eat only when hungry. Never eat just because the food is there and you want the pleasure of taste.
- Don't constantly and haphazardly snack.
- Ayurveda emphasizes a mealtime routine when food is consumed in a regular time the body knows when to expect food and in anticipation it secretes digestive enzymes to support the physiological function of digestion.
- Have a regular gap between meals three hours is recommended.
- Eat in a peaceful surrounding. Food is a energy source so unsettled emotions are likely to lead you to eat more quickly and to overeating.
- If you are upset do not eat. Wait till emotions are calmed down.
- Always sit down to eat. Food has to be honored a small prayer or grace will do wonders.

Developing Your Own Personalized Food Plan

For successful healthy outcome be it; Healthy eating weight loss, improve lipid profile, improved heart or brain health, better immunity, you need to make significant changes in life style choices. Consider these 7 strategies for success.

Change your perspective

For successful long-term health outcomes healthy eating must become a way of life. Adopt lifestyle changes by developing a strategy by taking an honest look at your daily routine, food habits, activity and exercise, mental habits etc.

- Try by working out a strategy by gradually changing habits and attitudes.
- Identify factors that sabotage efforts.
- Commit to never give up.
- Nobody can be perfect 100%, 100% of the time. If you slip, simply start afresh the next day. An 80:20 rule is also satisfactory.
- Always remember you are changing, it is a process and won't happen at once.

1. Write why you want to achieve the desired Goals and outcome.
   Try to be accountable for yourself by regularly recording and journaling your progress.
2. Make a commitment.
   It should be a long term one; you may need a lot of mental and physical energy to make the change. Be focused on your goals
3. Outline the outcomes you would like to achieve. Preferably write them down in a journal and tabulate them over a period of time.
   The outcomes could be objective (those that can be measured) like
   - Weight
   - Body measurements
   - Blood pressure
   - Lipid profile
   - Heart health
   - Blood sugar
   - Fasting A1C
   - All lab works
   - Physical fitness
   - Bone health

Some subjective outcomes are ones that cannot be measured but are important for you.i.e

- Mood and happiness

- Energy levels
- Activity levels
- Feeling of wellbeing etc

4. Outline your eating plan. – More plant based and as discussed earlier.
5. Use Herbs and spices and Enjoy healthy food for added health benefits.

   Don't give up on taste, satiety and satisfaction. Focus on ease of meal preparation, improve cooking skills, and enjoy a variety of food. Only remember to take care of quality of food, which should be fresh and wholesome.

   - Cut back on refined sugar (only maximum 1 tsp per day)
   - Cut back on refined carbohydrate and grains; replace with wholesome ancient grains.
   - Use healthy fats like Avocado oil, olive oil, coconut oil, and butter.
   - Avoid; processed meats and food, colas, tinned food eating in restaurants and monosodium glutamate a flavor enhancer used to make low quality food tastier.
   - Eat at least 4 servings of vegetables and maximum 2 servings of low glycemic fruit.
   - Drink 12 to 15 glasses of water the flavored water in the recipe section could be a delicious introduction to your lifestyle.

6. Get active and stay active

   You can lose weight, improve other outcomes, but the benefits of getting active and staying active cannot be undermined just a few;

   - It will boost your mood
   - Improve heart health and performance.
   - Improve flexibility, help with weight loss
   - Boost immunity

- Boost self-image

To start off aim to walk at least 30 mins /day on all days of week. Graduate to High intensity workouts, weights etc.

Sleep more

The relation of lack of sleep and many illnesses is being discovered by science. Try to sleep for 7 to 9 hours per day.

Most important you need to believe in the process and be positive and hopeful of the desired outcomes.

One of the causes of many diseases is stress. Stress causes a surge in cortisol secretion. It is well known cortisol raises insulin levels and is a major pathway for weight gain. Some of these winning strategies can help in winning the mind game

In today's world most of us are focused on the physical aspects of our bodies, how we look, how energetic we feel, we tend to neglect an very important dimension to detoxification and that is the emotional and mental aspect. So it is advised to do a mental and emotional fast

Emotional management

Aim to Connect with your body, mind and intellect. Food is a source of happiness for many and emotional eating is a huge problem. The book will be incomplete if we do not address the emotional part of personal management it a form of Behavioral cognitive therapy

Physical activity

Regular exercise is an excellent way to relieve stress and not only lowers cortisol levels but also helps by triggering secretion of serotonin and other feel good happy hormones. The endorphins secreted help in improving mood.

Find activities that you enjoy, going to the gym, dancing, a particular sport, be active and energetic the whole daylong.

Yoga, is a great way of balancing emotions by connecting the body, mind and intellect.

Have a massage to relax it is the most passive and easy way to relax.

Meditate!

Being calm relaxed and happy all the time is not all that simple, as there is often no escape from major every day causes of stress, pressure from people, unacceptable deadlines etc. Meditation relaxes the mind and is the best emotional management tool. You use guided meditation, mindfulness meditation, repeat a mantra or use candles. All of these do the same thing to your mind. Take the time off every day to reformat your mind, emotions and brain.

Accept stress is a side effect of modern life and one of the best ways to deal with it is Meditation.

Initiate a Mindful Happiness movement

We all need a strategy to help us be happy.

Happiness is attitude one needs to train oneself in. To some it comes naturally because of their genetical predisposition, natural temperament   but for most the mind needs to be trained in happiness by nurturing happiness. The mind needs a lot of practice with repeated reminders to stay in the happy state.

Start your 'happiness movement 'firstly increase your awareness with some facts regarding happiness, next develop an attitude of happiness.

Be a positive thinker; develop a mindful attitude of positivity may need behavior cognitive therapy for this.

Ask yourself what makes me happy? Mostly it is the simple things in life, which make most people happy; our friends, homes, and the beautiful world that we live in. Interestingly recent research has shown that happiness doesn't lie in materialism, but in modest living, gratitude and giving.

Research has also shown people have slowly realized that happiness may not lie in the relentless pursuit of hedonism. The key is to focus on simpler things; Relationships with family and friends. Contact with the nature.

Laugh and smile

Laughing has an instant effect on the feel good factor in the mind and body. Its surprising how you can feel immediately better by laughing and smiling, read jokes watch comedy films, repeat and narrate jokes to friends. If possible join a laughter club.

Be grateful - Gratitude is one of the biggest secrets to increase happiness. Practicing gratitude by silently counting on your blessings and especially by journaling them.

Be a giver one doesn't need to give expensive presents, most of the best gifts don't cost a lot; give a compliment, silent prayer or blessing.

Awaken the child in you

"We do not stop playing because we grow old. We grow old because we stop playing". Do childish things.

Choose happiness over being right. Remember that 'being happy and being right 'do not necessarily go hand in hand. When in a conflict situation, and in doubt, choose happiness over being right. This will change many things in your life.

Singing; if you are a shy person Sing when you are alone sing when you are driving. You can see negativity evaporate when you sing and dance.

Develop hobbies; Tap into your creative genius and find your "happy hobby".

Creativity is a great secret to happiness. If you can do creative things for a living even better. Cultivate your hobbies for happiness; Paint, draw, dance, sculpt, gardening, learn some craft, write, cook gourmet if your hobbies can help anyone even better volunteer.

Choose the people you hang out with happy people have fun around them and their ability to overcome challenges is higher than that of unhappy people. Negativity and positivity is infectious so hang around happy positive people, this will help you learn happiness

Invest in relationships

Accept every one, don't keep looking at their flaws and strive to be as less judgmental as possible. Be easy going. The worst attitude one can have is an attitude where one is easily offended this can only bring misery. Unfortunately these days many have developed an attitude where they are just waiting to be offended and seeking to be offended. Spend time with friends and family give and express unconditional love. Look at the positive side in every one it is a great way of nurturing love for people who matter most to you. Always remember the biggest causes of unhappiness are Health, Money and relationships, if you develop a strategy to balance all three you can be happy and satisfied.

Connect with community

Strive for social connectivity, as it is a great stress reliever. Be a part of a group or community, for many religion can provide this feeling. Give back to society by volunteering your help; a sure shot way of raising ones self-esteem.

Connect with the environment

Spend more time outdoor admiring the beautiful gifts of nature. Care for the environment by volunteer work.

It is most important to be focused at all times on your new lifestyle

CHAPTER 7.

RECIPES FOR SUCCESS USING REAL FOOD

Be ready to try and enjoy the delicious real food, food which is going to be your medicine. Many of the recipes have been collected from texts on Vedic nutrition.

Remember to put in all the information covered from chapter 5 and 6; try to locate and buy the highest quality local, organic non GMO food. Try to get pasture raised cage free, antibiotic free meat and wild caught sea food.

We understand one cannot follow 100% but the 80:20 rule is also quite good.

If cost is a concern, remember you are investing in good health and saving from medical bills ultimately. Savings will accumulate by:

- Not buying takeaways and saving from restaurant bills
- Reduced portion sizes
- Eating more plant based meals and less meats is a big saving
- Reduced medical bills in the long run. This is a huge saving
- Not to mention the increased energy, mental clarity and increased productivity having a potential to more income.

Feel free to customize the recipes to your tastes, for example if you don't like any herb or spices replace it. If you have an insulin resistance problem replace rice with low glycemic grains like buckwheat, Sorghum rice, quinoa.

Recipes for preparing probiotic rich, functional food

It is incredibly easy to make your own awesome, probiotic foods at home at the fraction of the cost of commercial preparations. Foods naturally ferment with naturally rich good bacteria under the right conditions; they can ferment into some delicious beverages, condiments and deserts. One of the major advantage is they will be free of all the undesired Toxic agents like food dyes, preservatives, flavor boosts, stabilizers and what not!

- Beverages –, Kefir Smoothies, Low carbohydrate functional smoothies, Kombucha tea
- Condiments – Pickles, Kimchi, Saukeraut, salsa, ketchup
- Fruit and vegetables
- Yoghurts – Probiotic Raitas
- Deserts – Cheese cake, gelato, shrikhand

Beverages

Basic Kefir
Ingredients

Two cups fresh milk any type of milk will work, including cow, goat, and pure coconut milk, raw milk is ideal, particularly goat milk. Traditionally raw milk is used for Kefir but Pasteurized milk will work too.

Kefir culture: available at health food stores /supermarkets. **You can use store bought kefir for culture.** Later keep using fresh culture from the kefir you have made.

Instructions

Warm the milk to a lukewarm temperature/ also boiling milk and letting it cool to a warm temperature test by being able to tolerate drops of milk over the back of your hand.

Next gently stir one tablespoon of culture preferably by a wooden spoon, set in yoghurt maker, or cover with a lid, and move to a warm location away from direct sunlight. This might be a cupboard, pantry, or darker side of the kitchen, placing it in a non-heated oven with oven Light also works.

Allow the mixture to ferment for a minimum of 24 hours. It is not advisable to go beyond 48 hours.

Kefir can be had in its natural form, or as a smoothie with fruit. .

Smoothies

Smoothies are a great way to combine kefir with just about any other nutritious food.

Use a combination of fresh and frozen fruit as you not only get a variety of fruit into your smoothie but also create a thick, ice-cold texture.

Use the basic smoothie formula and then move onto the many delicious combinations you'll find below. Whatever combination you choose, be sure to use fresh cultured kefir for the wonderful taste and living organisms it possesses.

- For 2 serving:
- 1 cup kefir
- 1/2 cup fresh fruit
- 1/2 cup frozen fruit
- Sweetener stevia/ truvia
- Flavorings: cardamom, cinnamon, vanilla, or mint

Functional smoothies: Add-ins Psyllium husk for its fiber, it swells to form a gel helps by suppressing hunger and leading to weight loss. Turmeric, powdered herbs or seaweeds, chia or flax seeds, flax or cod liver oil also can be added.

Blend all ingredients in a blender until smooth.

Strawberry Kefir and Banana Smoothie
Ingredients

- 1/2 large banana, broken into 6 chunks
- 1/2 cup sliced frozen strawberries
- 1 cup kefir
- 1 teaspoon honey

Instructions

Place your banana, strawberries and kefir into your blender

Blend for a couple of minutes or until smooth. Pour into a glass and enjoy

Blue berry Smoothie
Ingredients

- 3/4 cup kefir (plain)
- 1/2 cup frozen or fresh blueberries or blackberries
- ¼ tsp cinnamon powder
- 1 tbsp. honey/ stevia

Instructions

Blend in your blender and add honey or cinnamon if needed!

Mango, Kefir Smoothie
Ingredients

- 1 mango / 1 cup frozen mango slices
- 1 cup kefir

- 1/6 teaspoon cardamom powder
- 1 tbsp honey/ stevia to taste

Instructions
Blend until smooth.

Peach, orange Smoothie
Ingredients
- 1 cup plain kefir
- 1 cup fresh / frozen peaches
- 1 cup orange pulp/ orange juice
- 1/6 tsp vanilla powder
- 1-2 tablespoon honey

Instructions
Blend on high for 2 - 3 minutes and serve

Peachy-Ginger Smoothie
Ingredients
- Half cup Kefir
- Half cup fresh peaches
- Half cup frozen peaches
- 1 teaspoon minced slice of fresh ginger

Instructions
Blend on high for 2 - 3 minutes and serve

Green healthy Kefir
Ingredients
- 1 cup plain kefir or yogurt
- Half avocado
- 1/2 teaspoon chia seeds

- 1/2 cup, tightly packed, mixed baby greens, such as kale, red chard, and spinach
- Salt to taste
- 1 clove garlic
- Cumin seeds one fourth teaspoon

Instructions

Place all of the ingredients in a blender and blend at high speed for 1 minute or until smooth. Serve at once.

Peanut Butter-Banana Smoothie

Ingredients

- 1 frozen chopped banana
- 1 cup Kefir
- 2 tablespoons peanut butter
- 1 teaspoon honey/ stevia to taste

Instructions

Place all of the ingredients in a blender and blend at high speed for 1 minute or until smooth. Serve at once.

Merry -Berry Smoothie

Ingredients

- 1 cup kefir
- 1/2 cup frozen cherries
- 1/4 cup fresh / frozen blueberries
- 1/4 cup strawberries, or raspberries
- 1 teaspoon honey/ stevia to taste

Instructions

Place all of the ingredients in a blender and blend at high speed for 1 minute or until smooth. Serve at once.

Low carbohydrate smoothies

For diabetics, prediabetics, people on weight loss programs these functional recipes are useful as they are filling if psyllium husk is added hunger can be warded off as fiber swells and delays passage of food keeping one full for longer periods of time

Functional Food, Avocado Kefir Smoothie:

Ingredients

- and half cup kefir
- 1 avocado
- pods garlic
- salt,
- cumin /mint
- 1 tablespoon flaxseed or psyllium can be added to the smoothie if desired.

Instructions

Place all of the ingredients in a blender and blend at high speed for 1 minute or until smooth. Serve at once.

Cucumber Mint Smoothie

Ingredients

- and half cup kefir
- 1 peeled and sliced cucumber
- ¼ tsp roasted and ground cumin seeds
- Black salt to taste
- 1 green chilly
- 1tblspoon chopped mint leaves
- 1 tablespoon flaxseed or psyllium can be added to the smoothie if on weight loss program.

Instructions

Place all of the ingredients in a blender and blend at high speed for 1 minute or until smooth. Serve at once.

<u>Tomato celery Smoothie</u>

- 1 cup kefir
- 3 red frozen and peeled tomatoes
- 1 /2 peeled and sliced cucumber
- 6 inch sliced celery
- 1 tbsp. olive oil
- 1 tbsp. red wine vinegar
- 1 green chilly
- Salt to taste
- 2 pods garlic
- 1 tablespoon flaxseed or psyllium can be added to the smoothie if on weight loss program.

Instructions

Place all of the ingredients in a blender and blend at high speed for 1 minute or until smooth. Serve at once.

<u>Kale Smoothie</u>

- 1 cup kefir
- 1 cup packed deveined kale leaves
- 1 frozen and peeled tomato
- 6 inch sliced celery
- 1 tbsp. ginger/ 1 pod garlic
- Salt to taste
- 1 tablespoon flaxseed or psyllium can be added to the smoothie if on weight loss program .

Instructions

Place all of the ingredients in a blender and blend at high speed for 1 minute or until smooth. Serve at once.

Kanji
Ingredients
- 3 carrots cut in sticks
- 1 beet peeled cut in strips
- 1 teaspoon crushed mustard seeds
- 1/2 tsp red chili powder
- 1 tsp Kosher salt/ pickling salt
- 1 1/2 liter water

Instructions
Mix all the above ingredients. Cover with a lid or a muslin and keep the jars in the sun. Allow fermenting for 2-3 days until the drink becomes sour. Stir the mixture every day with a clean wooden spoon before placing in the sun.

Kombucha tea
Kombucha tea is a traditionally fermented sour tea. This method for continuous brewing ensures a consistent supply of kombucha tea, and is easy to maintain. For this kombucha, you'll need a kombucha starter culture, which you can find online. Now most health food store shelve Kombucha tea bags can be used for convenience.

Ingredients
- 2 tablespoons loose-leaf tea
- 1 cup organic white sugar
- 1 kombucha mother
- 1 cup kombucha tea from a previous batch

Instructions

Bring one quart of water to a boil. Turn off the heat, stir in tea and organic sugar. Continue stirring until the sugar is dissolved. Allow the tea to sit undisturbed until it cools to room temperature.

Strain the tea through a fine-mesh sieve into your continuous brew container. Stir in 3 quarts water. Add the kombucha mother and the kombucha tea to the container. Cover it loosely, and allow it to ferment about a week.

After a week, draw off up to one fourth of the kombucha, bottle it, and replace it with an equivalent amount of sweet tea. After the initial week of fermentation, you can draw off kombucha as frequently as you like - usually 1 to 3 times a week - as long as you replace it with an equivalent amount of tea.

Condiments –Kimchi, Saukeraut, Pickles, Salsa, Ketchup

Kimchi
Ingredients

- 1 (2-pound) Napa cabbage
- 1/2 cup kosher salt
- about 12 cups cold water, more as needed
- 8 ounces Daikon radish, peeled, and cut into 2-inch matchsticks
- 4 medium scallions, ends trimmed, cut into 1-inch pieces (use all parts)
- 1/3 cup Korean red pepper powder
- ¼ cup fish sauce
- 1/4 cup peeled and minced fresh ginger (from about a 2-ounce piece)
- 1 tablespoon minced garlic cloves (from 6 to 8 medium cloves)
- 2 teaspoons Korean salted shrimp, minced (optional)

- 1 1/2 teaspoons granulated sugar

Instructions

1Cut the cabbage in half lengthwise, then crosswise into 2-inch pieces, discarding the root end. Place in a large bowl, sprinkle with the salt, and toss with your hands until the cabbage is coated. Add enough cold water to just cover (about 12 cups), making sure the cabbage is submerged (it's okay if a few leaves break the surface). Let sit for 4-6 hours.

- Place a colander in the sink, drain the cabbage, and rinse with cold water. Gently squeeze out the excess liquid and transfer to a medium bowl. Set aside.
- Mix all the ingredients until you get a paste. Add to the cabbage and toss with your hands until evenly combined and the cabbage is thoroughly coated with the mixture.
- Pack the mixture tightly into a clean 2-quart or 2-liter glass jar with a tight fitting lid and seal the jar.
- Let sit in a cool, dark place for 24 hours (the mixture may bubble). Open the jar to let the gases escape, then reseal and refrigerate at least 48 hours before eating. (Kimchi is best after fermenting about 1 week.) Refrigerate for up to 1 month.

Saukeraut

Ingredients

- 5 lbs. of cabbage
- 1/4 cup Kosher or Pickling Salt
- Large Jar /Container needs to be glass
- 2 large plastic zip-lock bags

Instructions

Sanitize containers/ utensils in dishwasher or with boiling water

Remove outer leaves and cores from cabbage

Thinly slice cabbage

Mix 4 tbsp. salt with cabbage and let stand in a bowl to wilt .

When juice starts to form on cabbage/salt mixture, pack tightly into bottle using sanitized spoon or clean hands

Repeat this until cabbage is within about 4-5 inches of top of container

Pack down until water level rises above cabbage and all cabbage is entirely submerged

If there is not enough liquid to cover cabbage, make a brine with 1½ tbsp. salt in 1 quart of water. Add cooled brine to the jar until all cabbage is completely covered

Once cabbage is submerged, fill a food-grade freezer bag with brine

Place brine-filled bag on top of cabbage in jar making sure that it touched all edges and prevents air from reaching cabbage.

Cover jar with plastic wrap and cloth or towel. tie tightly.

Place jar in an area that will be between 70 and 75 degrees.

Fermentation will begin within a day and take 3-5 weeks depending on temperature.

After 3 weeks, check for desired tartness.

Once fermented, it can be eaten right away, frozen or canned according to your canner's instructions.

Probiotic Green Tomatillo Salsa

Ingredients

- 1 lb. Tomatillos
- 1 lb. Green Tomatoes
- 1 spring onion
- 5 cloves of minced garlic
- Half cup Fresh Cilantro to taste (I use 1/2 cup or more)
- 1 lemon, juiced
- 2 Tbsp. sea salt
- ¼ tsp each oregano, chilly, pepper, and cumin

- 1 tbsp. minced jalapeno pepper
- 1/2 cup fermented whey (refer to recipe in following pages)

Instructions

Chop tomatoes, peppers, onion and cilantro and mince garlic.

Toss all ingredients into large glass bowl

Add the juice of the lemon and lime

salt and spices to taste and whey

Mix thoroughly

Pour into mason jars and cap tightly.

Leave on the counter for approximately 2 days.

Refrigerate

Red Salsa

- 4 cup red tomatoes, peeled, chopped deseeded and drained
- 1 cup chopped onions
- 1/2 cup green bell peppers
- 1 /2cup jalapeno pepper, chopped
- 4 cloves garlic minced
- 1 teaspoons cumin
- 1teaspoons pepper
- 1 tsp sugar
- 4 tsp sea salt
- 1 (12 ounce) can tomato paste
- ½ cup whey

Directions:

This is a chunky salsa so if you want a smoother salsa cut your veggies into smaller pieces.

Mix all ingredients

Place in warm dark place for 24- 48 hours

<u>**Whey and probiotic cream cheese**</u>

Homemade whey is used for fermenting vegetables and condiments
Preparation is quite simple

Ingredients

- 1 liter container of probiotic store/ homemade yoghurt/ kefir
- Cheese cloth /thin towel
- Glass container

Instructions

Place cheese cloth over a strainer
Empty yoghurt /Kefir
Tie the loose ends of the cloth
Collect the strained liquid in a glass bowl
The liquid is the whey and the solid thick cream is cream cheese in the desert section this is an important ingredient.

<u>**Probiotic Chili sauce can prepare Red /yellow/ green / orange**</u>

Ingredients

- 200 gr chilies, red/yellow/ green stems removed if you like it to be extra hot use hot chilies
- 3 cloves of garlic
- 8 gr sea salt
- water to cover
- half cup raw apple cider vinegar

Instructions

First cut off the stems of the chilies. For mild sauce you can remove the seeds of the chilies as well.

Roughly chop chilies and add them to a clean jar (this is the jar in which they will ferment so make sure it fits them all and also water to cover).

Add sea salt and water just enough to cover, plus and extra half cm.

Stir using, cover the jar with some cheesecloth (or a paper towel) and secure it with an elastic band.

Place the jar in a cool dark place in the pantry, away from direct sunlight.

Every other day or so check your chilies to see if any white mold forms on top. If it does, simply remove it with a clean spoon and give your chili mix another stir. Cover and place it back in the pantry.

To see if fermentation is taking place, check for tiny bubbles forming either on top or through the chili mix.

Fermentation is complete anywhere between 4 to 6 weeks, depending on temperature.

After fermenting the chilies, add the entire mixture to a blender and whiz it up for few seconds until completely pureed and as fine as possible.

Strain this mix through a fine sieve and press it with a spoon to get as much juice out as possible. If too thick add apple cider vinegar.

Keep refrigerated until finished.

Probiotic Ketchup
Ingredients

- Three 6-oz jars/cans of <u>tomato paste</u>
- 1/3 cup <u>raw honey</u>
- 3 Tb raw <u>apple cider vinegar</u>
- 3 small garlic cloves, pressed
- 6 Tb <u>sauerkraut</u> juice or whey
- 2 1/4 tsp <u>finely ground salt</u>
- ½ teaspoon pinch <u>cayenne pepper</u>

Directions

Combine all ingredients in a glass bowl with a wooden spoon.Stir well to combine

Ensure that the top of the ketchup is at least 1-inch below the top of the jar(s).

Using a clean cloth or paper towel, wipe the top of the jar above the ketchup clean.

Put lid on jar and leave at room temperature for 3 days; then transfer to the refrigerator.

Herbal and Spiced Teas

Most of the health retreats at the Ashrams and spas in India, rely on fasting with herbal teas for detoxification since centuries. Healing by the medicinal herbs focuses on the liver and gut health rest whole body healing follows. The warm tea fill up the stomach fooling it that there is some food, and that helps by keeping hunger at bay. Most ashrams avoid green tea as it has caffeine, however Spas do allow green tea

- 1.Curcumin Tea Recipe
- Curcumin tea is quick and easy to prepare.
- 1/2 teaspoon of ground turmeric or 1 inch of freshly grated turmeric.
- 2 cups of water.
- Pinch of Black pepper is said to improve bioavailability of turmeric.

Preparation:

Bring water to a boil, and then reduce to simmer. Add ground turmeric and continue to simmer for approximately five to ten minutes. Add a dash of freshly ground black pepper. Use mesh strainer or cheesecloth to strain. Can be used as is or add any additional desired flavors, like honey, lemon juice, etc. Can be combined with green tea also.

Variations: Turmeric along with ginger can prepared. If one is not fasting milk and honey can be added and had during the eating window

Curcumin tea is recommended twice a day.

Ginger tea

- 2 cms piece of Grated ginger
- To prepare the tea pour hot water over the tea let it sit for 3to 4 minutes strain and drink

Green tea with ginger

Grate 1 cm piece of ginger. Add 1 teaspoon or a bag of green tea
Pour Boiling water over the tea let it seep for 2-3 mins strain and enjoy

Green tea with mint

Add a teaspoon of dried or fresh mint to 1 teaspoon or a bag of green tea.
Pour Boiling water over the tea let it steep for 2-3 mins strain and enjoy
Spiced Masala green tea
Grind 1 star aniseed, 1-inch cinnamon, 5 cardamoms, 2 cloves, and 4 peppercorns Add a pinch of this to your usual green tea.
For those avoiding caffeine add half teaspoon in hot water to 1fourt of a tsp of spice strain and enjoy masala tea.
This is a special detoxifying herbal tea recipe given to me by one of my sister from one of India's famous Ashram in Mount Abu

Morning herbal tea:

½ tsp coriander seeds
½ tsp cumin seeds
½ tsp fennel seeds
4-5 leaves mint
¼ tsp cinnamon powder
1/4 tsp oregano seeds

Boil all these in two cups water. Filter it when one-cup water is left. Put 2-3 drops of fresh lemon juice. You can put a little honey if you are not in the fasting window.

There are a whole lot of Herbal teas described in Ayurveda according to Dosa type.

Liver cleansening herbal teas for detoxification

Liver detox tea

A maximum liver detox prepare a mixture of 1 oz each the following dried herbs

- 1 oz Milk thistle
- 1 oz Dandelion root
- 1oz Licorice root
- 1 oz Wild yam root
- 1 oz Barberry bark
- 1 oz tanners oak bark.
- Prepare the dry mix of above herbs by coarsely crushing them. Store in an airtight container for daily use.
- Soak one tablespoon of the mix with 8 oz warm water leave to soak overnight and have it in the morning.

Teas for Insulin Resistance

- Herbal Tea mix
- 2 oz coriander seeds
- 2 oz ground turmeric
- 2 oz dried ginger
- 2 oz fenugreek seeds.

Crush these to a very coarse mix, add 2 tablespoon of this to 30 oz of water let it sit overnight, then bring to boil, let it simmer for 5-10 minutes strain and drink 2 cups of this herbal tea daily.

Citrus Tea Mix

Mix

- 1 oz Dried Orange rind
- 1 Oz dried lemon rind
- 1 oz Dried Grapefruit rind
- 4 oz dried lemon grass
- Coarsely dry grind and store in airtight container/ jar
- Pour 1-cup boiling water on 1 tbs of mix let it steep for 3-5 mins before consuming

Masala Chai

Mix the following dry ingredients

- 8 oz black tea leaves
- 1 oz cardamom pods lightly bruised
- 1 oz cinnamon sticks broken to 1 cm pieces
- ½ oz Cloves
- 3 Star Anise
- 1 nutmeg coarsely ground
- 1 tsp ground dry ginger
- Mix above and store in an airtight jar. Can be used for many variations as desired

Black masala chai:

Pour 1 cup of boiling water over 1 tsp of above chai mix, steep for 4-5 mins. Strain and enjoy black.

Chai Latte:

Mix can be used for Chai latte if one is not fasting – Boil 1 cup milk add 1 heaped tsp mix to the boiling milk add 1 tsp honey for the chai latte.

Turmeric Chai latte:

Can be made as regular Chai latte with addition of 1 tsp of freshly crushed turmeric root for a boutique style chai latte.

Bitter Mellon Tea

Research has now shown that Bitter melon has properties to regenerate the beta cells in the pancreas in animal model. For centuries Ayurveda has been recommending bitter melon for diabetics. In Asia it is widely consumed. A tea can be prepared by pouring boiling water over 4-5 slices of the melon, steeping for 5 mins. Also the melon can be sliced, dried and stored for convenience and used as desired.

Sacred Basil tea (Tulsi tea)

This is a popular Herbal tea used in India. Sacred basil is dried and steeped in boiling water; strained and consumed often it is mixed with ginger. This tea is said to balance the cortisol levels in the body

Cool drinks

Consume 12 - 15 glasses of filtered water per day

Flavored water

Lemon water:

Add 4 Slices of lemon to 2 liters of filtered water with ice. Drink throughout the day. 1 tsp Apple cider vinegar can be also added to the water

Peach Water:

Add slices of 1 peach to 3 liters of water

Coriander, ginger and lime water: Add a2 sprigs of coriander leaves along with slices of lime to 2 liter of water

Apple Water:

Add slices of 1 Apple to 3 liters of water

Lemon grass water:

Add 1 root and leaves of lemon grass, 1 tbsp apple cider vinegar to 3 liters of water

Passion fruit water:

Add one passion fruit to 4 liters of cold water

Cucumber water:

1 cucumber, juice of half lime, 1 cup cilantro, half teaspoon apple cider vinegar pinch of rock salt and pepper.

Broths

<u>Clear Vegetable Broth</u>

- To 4- 6 liters of filtered water
- 1 large onion
- 1 garlic
- 2 tomatoes
- 1 cup chopped celeriac
- 4 sticks of celery
- 2 parsnips
- 2 leeks
- 2 tbsp coriander seeds

- 1 teaspoon pepper corns
- 1tspoon cumin seeds
- 1 teaspoon turmeric
- 1 teaspoon fenugreek seeds
- 2 tsp Himalayan salt.
  Boil for 2-4 hours strain add few drops of lemon juice just before drinking.

Chicken Broth

To 6- 8 liters of filtered water add 2 pound chicken bones/ 1 whole chicken , 2 tbs apple cider vinegar, 1 large onion, 1 garlic, 4 sticks of celery, 2 leeks, 1 stick lemon grass, 2 tbsp coriander seeds, 1 teaspoon pepper corns, 1tspoon cumin seeds and 1 teaspoon turmeric, 1 teaspoon fenugreek seeds. 2 tsp Himalayan salt. Boil and then let it simmer for 4 to 6 hours strain add few drops of lemon juice just before drinking.

Soups
- 1.Vegetable soup
- 2 cups cabbage
- 2 tomatos
- 2 cloves garlic
- 1-cup French beans
- ½ cup scallions
- ½ teaspoon fenugreek
- ½ teaspoon turmeric
- ½ teaspoon cumin
- ½ teaspoon cayenne /black pepper
- Boil all the ingredients till vegetables are soft and then blend in blender

Celery soup

- 2 cups chopped celery root/ celeriac
- 2 clove garlic
- 2-stalk celery stalk
- Pinch of rock salt
- ½ cup cilantro
- ¼ cup almond milk
  Boil and blend all the ingredients except almond milk and cilantro add while blending

Herbal Red lentil soup

- 2 cups seeded and chopped tomatoes
- 1 cup chopped French beans
- 3 tablespoon red lentil
- 1 cup chopped okra
- 1 cup chopped carrots
- 3 cups water
- 2 cloves garlic
- 1-inch ginger
- ½ cup chopped onions
- ½ teaspoon fenugreek
- ½ teaspoon cayenne pepper/black pepper
- 2 cloves
- 1/3-teaspoon cinnamon
- ½ teaspoon turmeric
- ½ teaspoon cumin
- 10-12 Sweet neem leaves (Curry leaves)
- ½ cup finely chopped cilantro
  Boil /pressure cook/slow cook all ingredients except the cilantro add cilantro before serving

Broccoli soup

- 2 cups chopped broccoli
- ½ teaspoon butter
- 1-cup water
- 2 cloves garlic
- ½ cup onions
- Pinch of rock salt
- Pinch of pepper
- ½ cup almond milk
- 1 cup parsley

Sauté broccoli in butter and cook, add rest of the ingredients, except parsely and almond milk. Which are to be added when blending.

Cauliflower soup

- 2Cups chopped cauliflower
- ½ teaspoon butter
- 2-cup water
- ½ inch ginger
- Pinch of rock salt
- Pinch of pepper
- 1-cup cilantro
- ½ teaspoon fenugreek
- ½ teaspoon cayenne pepper/black pepper
- 2 cloves garlic
- ½ teaspoon turmeric
- ½ teaspoon cumin
  Sauté cauliflower in butter and cook, add rest of the ingredients, except coriander and milk. Which are to be added when blending

Brussels sprouts

- 2 cup Brussels sprouts
- 2 cups water
- ½ teaspoon butter
- 1 cm ginger
- 1-teaspoon miso paste
- Dash of sesame oil.
  Sauté Brussels sprouts in butter
- Add rest of the ingredients
- Blend

<u>**Spinach and Almond soup**</u>

- 2 cups frozen spinach
- ½ cup frozen fenugreek leaves
- 1-cup water
- ½ cup onion
- 2 cloves garlic
- Pinch of salt
- ½ cup Almond milk
  Boil all the ingredients except Almond milk
  Blend adding Almond milk

<u>**Khichadi**</u>
Ingredients:
- 1 cup split yellow mung dahl beans
- ¼ – ½ cup long grain white or white basmati rice
- 1 tbsp fresh ginger root
- 1 tsp each: black mustard seeds, cumin, and turmeric powder
- ½ tsp each: coriander powder, fennel and fenugreek seeds

- 3 cloves
- 3 bay leaves
- cloves garlic
- 1 large tomato
- 7-10 cup water
- ½ tsp salt (rock salt is best)
- 1 small handful chopped fresh cilantro leaves
- 2 cups mixed frozen vegetables
  Wash split yellow mung beans and rice together until water runs clear.

In a pre-heated large pot, dry roast all the spices (except the bay leaves) on medium heat for a few minutes. This dry roasting will enhance the flavor. Alternately the spices can be tempered in oil.
Add dahl and rice and stir, coating the rice and beans with the spices.
Add all the rest ingredients.
Add water and bay leaves and bring to a boil.
Boil for 10 minutes.
Turn heat to low, cover pot, and continue to cook until dahl and rice become soft (about 30-40 minutes).
The cilantro leaves can be added just before serving.
Add a teaspoon of ghee.

Savory crepes
- ¼ cup Amaranth flour/ sorgum flour/millet flour
- 1 egg
- 1 teaspoon avacado oil
- Salt and pepper to taste
- Spinach 2 cups
- 2 table spoon goat cheese
- Method

- Blend the egg amaranth flour, oil salt and pepper.
- Spread thinly on a flat non stick pan
- Dot with butter
- When roasted and cooked add spinach and cheese
- Fold and serve hot.

9 781796 593013